THE

RESET

PLAN

Lose the **Secrets**
Lose the **Excuses**
Lose the **Weight**

BY

SHANNA FERRIGNO

ISBN-10: 0-692-87107-1
ISBN-13: 978-0-692-87107-2

Editing by Sherry Granader & Julia Todd
Cover & interior design by Charlotte Shih
Nutrition consulting by Kim Braniff
Photography by Jon Dow

Printed in the United States of America
First Printing March 2017

Published by Shanna Ferrigno
www.TheResetPlanBook.com

DEDICATION

"There is no need to be perfect to inspire others.
Let people get inspired by how you deal with your imperfections."
— Robert Tew

The Reset Plan is dedicated to everyone who decides to take that
first step towards Focusing, Investing and Taking Action to something
greater in their lives. You'll never know how many lives you are changing
by being brave enough to start a conversation that matters, but it all starts
with facing your truth and learning how to love yourself.

TABLE OF CONTENTS

FOREWORD

I am so proud of my daughter Shanna. I'm inspired by the courage, determination, and motivation she used to transform herself from an overweight kid into an elite athlete. I've been thrilled to watch her grow as a personal trainer and a successful businesswoman, and to see how she is using her life and skills to develop our business, Ferrigno FIT, which she continues to take to new levels of success. I can't say I'm surprised because from the time Shanna was a little girl, she was always happy to help people in need. Health and fitness have played a defining role in her life and career, as they have in mine, and it has been a joy to see her help others experience the difference being truly FIT can make in all aspects of their lives.

Shanna is a multi talented person, a hard worker. She is also an effective advocate for promoting fitness and educating people of all walks of life to maintain a health and fitness lifestyle. She gets great results from her clients and our business because she understands that no matter what challenges we face, improving our health will help us improve all aspects of our lives. Shanna also knows that life's struggles are never over and we must find sustainable solutions to use on a daily basis. We all have an inner Hulk that is ready to sabotage our best intentions. We can't completely remove this part of ourselves; we can only learn to quiet, control, and manage those negative influences. With enough strength and determination it can be done, and *The Reset Plan* will give people the tools to get started, both physically and emotionally.

It is a gift to see my daughter help others become stronger, stay FIT, and become better people. I can't wait to help Shanna share her message and strategies with readers, and will make myself available for promotion of *The Reset Plan* in any way that is helpful, including through social media, television, or personal appearances with her. When readers see how healthy their lives, relationships, and bodies can be after following her guidance, they'll wonder how it was they ever lived any other way.

With wishes for good all around health,

Lou Ferrigno
(Proud Father)

PREFACE

The Reset Plan: Lose the Secrets, Lose the Excuses, Lose the Weight is different than other diet books. This is not a gimmicky plan promising extreme weight loss; it is a safe, sane, and holistic plan to lose weight in a way that lasts. *The Reset Plan* works because it provides detailed plans for food and exercise in the context of getting you to understand why you have let yourself get out of control in the first place. After analyzing common "secrets" my clients — and I — have carried and used as excuses to keep from optimizing overall health, I offer specific advice and course-correction for those who are struggling. I promise to offer you a motivating and enthusiastic voice of a coach who is empathetic but does not accept excuses.

I consider myself upbeat, fun, accessible, and, most of all, straightforward about helping you lose weight. We'll look at the big picture and also get down to micro-level tips about how to make real, sustainable changes. *The Reset Plan* goes deep into a discussion of the psychology of shame and food addiction so that you can attain and maintain true fitness. The tone is not at all academic — I hope to appeal to anyone who likes the direct, tough-love style.

By looking at your weight loss journey in the context of achieving fitness, happiness, and success, it is my hope that this book will be not only intriguing to you but will also help you maximize your potential.

Growing up as the daughter of a famous actor in California and still training clients in that environment, I have realistic and down-to-earth expectations for your fitness journey, in terms of cost and time. *The Reset Plan* is a flexible guide for anyone who may have tried many other diets and either failed, or succeeded but then gained it all back, and still has weight to lose. *The Reset Plan* will explain why other diets didn't work and give you tools and inspiration to make permanent change.

The robust market for weight loss books and the increasing numbers of overweight Americans make it clear there is room for a new approach. *The Reset Plan* helps you take a deeper look at how you got where you are and is also unapologetic and practical about showing you how to lose the weight. I offer a voice some may find a bit unusual, with a proven combination of compassionate acceptance and hardball motivation, partnered with a weight loss plan to help you lose weight and keep it off.

The Reset Plan is a life, diet, and fitness plan... it is not a therapy session. Each week of this plan is structured around an excuse I hear frequently from my clients and friends: I call these the "Top Ten Lies We Tell Ourselves." I use each "lie" as a jumping-off point to introduce a new element or stage of *The Reset Plan* program. While the sections are based on commonly addressed issues, the plan itself is not dependent on you having one particular problem as opposed to another. If people recognize themselves in the various examples and descriptions, however, they will find practical advice for confronting whichever excuse they tend to use.

The goal of this book is to understand how and why I have developed *The Reset Plan*, and show it is possible to change, succeed, slide backwards, and recover; my own journey is proof. The connection between physical fitness and emotional fitness is ignored in most books about weight loss, and my story illustrates their relationship. Part of my authority as a trainer and coach comes from my own experience, which gives me the ability to identify with my clients: I have been where they are, and am proof of what is possible. We introduce the idea of letting go of the lies that may undermine the best intentions around diet and exercise, which forms the foundation of *The Reset Plan*.

The Reset Plan is designed to improve your health, help you enjoy better fitness, and lose weight through a combination of diet and exercise. It also explicitly addresses the psychological obstacles people use to avoid taking care of themselves.

I know people get excited about a drastic plan of action promising immediate results. The problem is that changes, if they occur at all, usually don't stick, and the "dieter" is back where they started and feeling like a failure. The *Obesity Research and Clinical Practice* journal published a study which showed it is harder for adults today to maintain the same weight as those twenty to thirty years ago, even when they were maintaining the same levels of exercise and food intake.

There are three main reasons why it is harder for adults to stay lean today. First and foremost, people are exposed to more chemicals than ever before that alter hormonal processes in the body. Substances in food packaging, pesticides, and flame-retardants tweak the way our bodies gain and maintain weight.

Secondly, the use of prescription drugs has grown dramatically since the 1980s to include antidepressants and other medications linked to weight gain. Finally, it is now well-known that certain types of gut bacteria can make a person more prone to gaining weight. Many people eat more meat than ever before and unfortunately, those animals have been treated with antibiotics and growth hormones in order to promote growth of the animal. When we eat animals treated with such hormones and antibiotics, it changes the bacteria in our gut and adds up over time. Considering also how artificial sweeteners have been added to the mix, you can see how our food supply has changed significantly.

The behaviors that help people lose weight are pretty general, but can be overwhelming to make all at once. I have found most clients do best when they make changes in stages by slowly upgrading their food choices and movement plans over time, which is why *The Reset Plan* introduces new challenges during each seven-day period rather than asking people to dive into drastic changes.

My experience with clients has also helped me understand that sustainable weight loss is only achieved by understanding the specific personal reasons why you are gaining weight in the first place. Based on my clients' successes, *The Reset Plan* frames each seven-day period within a discussion of a common problem faced by people struggling with weight: I call them "lies" or excuses we tell ourselves, and use each one to bridge into the food and movement upgrades people will make during the next seven day period.

INTRODUCTION

I help people transform their bodies and their lives, which is a kickass way to make a living. After training hundreds of clients, I co-founded my business, Ferrigno FIT, in order to develop and implement fitness programs that are truly effective at helping people reach their goals, whether they are around weight loss, bodybuilding, or other kinds of wellness. FIT stands for Focus, Invest, and Take Action, and *The Reset Plan* will show you how to use all three tools to make dramatic improvements to your health: **Focus** on what you want out of life. **Invest** in yourself. **Take Action** to transform into your true potential.

The reason our programs work is because we don't only focus on the weight or physical training of the people who come to us for help. The first thing I tell my clients is they have got to be honest with themselves.

Creating sustainable lifestyle change requires a commitment to your own mental health and a willingness to be the honest auditor of your life, which means confronting your secrets.

We all have secrets. Every person I have ever worked with has shame and embarrassment of some kind, often around more than one issue. Many people numb the pain and stress of keeping secrets by self-sabotaging with food. If this is you and *The Reset Plan* helps you to confront and address the secrets honestly and interrupt this behavior pattern, I promise: you will lose weight if you need to lose weight. You will become more physically FIT, be in a better mood, and be a happier person. If it sounds too good to be true, do the hard work and find out.

How do I know this might be you? Hundreds of clients have trained with me during the last decade and I know food addiction does not discriminate. Our reasons for overeating may be diverse: we use food to bond with family and friends or to be accepted, we may finish everything on our plates even when we are not hungry in order to be respectful or to not waste.

Some of us are eating to avoid feeling things that are uncomfortable.

Many of us are uneducated about basic facts of nutrition, portion size, and our bodies. The common theme among the people I have worked with who battle with food is that embarrassing habits or occasional indulgences turned into a more dangerous kind of shame: they hide what they eat from family, friends and colleagues, and develop massive denial about their behavior.

Many people I work with who struggled with food believed or pretended that the food they were overeating didn't exist when no one was watching them. Another frequent little lie is to not "count" or notice the food eaten outside of regular mealtimes: the taste while cooking, the snack in the car, the sample at the bakery, the leftovers while cleaning up. There are so many opportunities to consume food mindlessly, and the mistake so many of us make is not in taking them, but rather in failing to be accountable to ourselves about the choices we make and the reasons we make them. The kind of denial leading to poor habits can run deep on the inside but the truth of it always is clear on the outside.

Do I sit people down during our first session together and demand they tell me their deepest secrets? Of course I don't. Am I saying that in order to be fit you need to reveal your dark side to the world? Not at all — but you have to be brutally honest with *yourself* and know that there will be people who will be there to hear you and help you when you are ready to share your truth and commit to change.

You can start small. Educate yourself about healthy behaviors. Start moving. Make changes in your diet. There are a lot of tools in this book and you can explore them in bits and pieces and see how it feels. To see real and lasting results, you must stick with these new habits since that's where most diet and exercise plans will fail you — as you probably know, if you've been down this road before.

Can I promise you that you will lose a certain number of pounds in a certain number of days if you use every tool and follow every rule in this book? No. What your goals are, and how long it will take you to reach them, is completely personal and depends on the commitments and changes you're willing to make.

The paths we each need to take to reach our goals are unique. Respect your own energy. The people who are going to make lasting changes will know when they are ready to go deeper and move forward on the journey.

Helping people evaluate when and how to push harder is part of my role as a trainer and a lifestyle coach. I've had to learn how to evaluate when someone is ready to try a new exercise, increase the amount of weight they can lift, or the number of repetitions they can do. Ideally, you want a client to be challenged, but to an appropriate degree so they aren't set up to fail. Everyone has different targets that are constantly moving, especially as people start making positive changes in their lives.

Use this book to challenge yourself the way I might if we could train together in person, where you will Focus, Invest, and Take Action to become as FIT as you have ever been in your life – both mentally and physically.

How did I learn this? I learned it the hard way. I have been grappling with my own embarrassment around food and body issues since childhood, which transformed into shame and self-damaging behavior. Only now can I say I truly feel beautiful and worthy, and it is my mission to make you feel the same way about yourself.

I grew up in Santa Monica, California. My father, Lou Ferrigno, was already well-known for being a world-class bodybuilder by the time I was born, having won Mr. Universe and Mr. America titles. He was also famous for playing the Incredible Hulk. Dad was primarily acting during the earlier part of my childhood, playing not just the Hulk in different television shows and movies, but other memorable roles as well, including Hercules.

I didn't completely understand how he made his living but remember knowing other people thought my father was special. He and my mother Carla, who manages my father's career, worked hard to provide a privileged life for my brothers and me. It was much more comfortable than the ones they had been given as children.

People always used to ask me, "What is it like to have the Incredible Hulk as your father?"

I never knew how to answer that question. I grew up feeling my dad was important. People seemed to like him and he would dress up as a green monster for work. Sometimes I worried kids wanted to come over to our house in order to hang out with him, not to play with me, because he was on television. When I was very young, I noticed he unintentionally intimidated some kids too, due to his size and his voice, which is affected by his childhood hearing loss. Once, when I was in kindergarten, he answered our front door and a little boy was standing on our front steps. He had come over to play but looked up at him and just burst into tears of terror.

Later in my childhood, I also watched my father stand on stage with a fake tan wearing Speedos, to pose and have his body be critiqued by judges. Our family would travel to different competitions around the world with him and that could be hard to watch. Sometimes, my dad would become emotional when he lost, or even came in second place. Even though I was developing mixed feelings about his job, and about watching him compete in the first place, I hated to see him lose.

The weird messages I was absorbing about the importance of the body were also messing with my head.

I was a ten-pound baby. As a young child, I had a sort of adorable Italian meatball type of body. In other words, I was never the skinny girl when I was growing up; nor did I consider myself to be especially pretty. Physically, I have always taken after my father's heartier side of the family. My mother, although she struggled with her weight as a child, was (and is) a beautiful, very petite blonde. As a little girl, I remember wishing I were graced with her tiny frame and blonde hair.

Even today, although I'm happy with the way I look, you will hear me joke that my mother always looks like she is entering a beauty pageant and I look like the one running it. My mother knew I was insecure about my looks as a kid; she tried her best to be reassuring and to make me feel beautiful and worthy. It worked for a while. I wasn't terribly self-conscious about my looks during my early childhood because my parents always made me feel accepted and beautiful.

And yet, when I was ten years old, I was 5'4", weighed 176 pounds and wore a size 36 in men's pants. Despite my parents always being health conscious, they never told me I was ugly, heavy, or overweight. Kids at school and some of my father's colleagues in the entertainment industry started to give me that message loud and clear, though. My family was walking a red carpet at the Emmy Awards that year, and my parents' publicist looked me up and down and suggested it might be best for me to step out of the photograph when we stopped to pose. My parents told her of course we would do no such thing, but I remember looking up at them and registering pity on their faces. It was shaming.

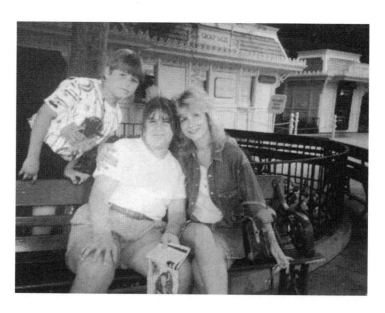

I knew I had a problem, and even though I was starting to understand from my classmates they didn't find me pretty, I still thought I had a secret.

I would go to the local drug store under the auspice of needing to buy a friend a birthday gift. If I really needed a birthday gift, I was searching for the cheapest possible present and card because I knew if I spent less money on my friend's birthday gift, I could buy what I really came to get: sugar. Sometimes I didn't truly have any reason to be at the store but I always had a story. I lied about having to get sweets for bake sales, science projects, school fairs, and hunger drives. You read that correctly: I said I needed to buy food to donate to a hunger drive.

Under whatever cover story I had devised, I would hit the candy aisle and grab my usual: three Snickers bars, one Almond Joy, one pack of gum (not sugar-free) and a giant handful of Jolly Ranchers. I remember always trying to pay quickly so I would not be seen — and sometimes I threw in two lollipops or something at the last minute if I thought that the usual cashier wouldn't remember, and judge, my basket of purchases.

I was a smart and self-conscious kid. Sometimes I didn't actually have to tell a made-up story to anyone to explain myself, but I was making the stories up for me, just in case. It was clear to me my parents would disapprove of my candy-buying and bingeing, and I was paranoid that friends, relatives, or neighbors would witness me executing my secret plans. I knew I was doing something "wrong" and I felt ashamed.

Guilt and embarrassment were driving forces in my life. I schemed about how to avoid exposure and planned on how to lie when I couldn't avoid it. Both were a part of my secret. Looking back, the saddest part of my "candy plan" was the fact that it was a plan. I planned those lies and cover stories about a friend's birthday, just in case I had to give a reason for why I was buying candy again. The shame of that was more profound and just as damaging, in its own way, as the actual overeating. There were secret consequences from my behavior as well, like the constant rashes on my inner thighs created by the skin on my legs rubbing together when I walked. I would hide my rash cream under my bed, next to my secret candy stash.

My parents, who are both supportive and amazing people, are not responsible for my weight gain, and I have always felt very clear about that. But, as adults, we have discussed this period of my childhood and why they "allowed" me to get so big and eat things I knew were bad for me. Their answer makes sense to me. They knew what they put down on the table for us to eat for breakfast and dinner were healthy choices. They also had both come to terms with their own weight issues, and knew they could fundamentally best lead by example.

Finally, after my very early childhood, they knew they could not ultimately control what I ate or how much I ate and so were determined not to create a power struggle over it.

Food can be as addictive as a drug, and issues around food are similar, in some ways, to issues with alcohol and substance dependency. I read a lot about alcohol addiction when I developed the Incredibly FIT program because I knew it was critical to address underlying issues in order to help clients create lasting success around food and fitness.

In some ways, food is actually is more problematic than drugs or other things people can become dependent on because food can't be completely eliminated from your life. We need to eat for energy, and it is possible to overeat even healthy foods that have redeeming nutritional qualities.

Food is also a pleasure that is an important part of living a good life. It is available everywhere and so can be the easiest — and often cheapest — numbing agent of choice to locate when we have the impulse to reach out for that kind of comfort. My parents understood all this and let me be, trusting that they were going to be the solution when I decided I needed one. And they were. But changes in my family, I have also come to understand, were part of my problem.

My weight gain coincided with my father's return to professional bodybuilding in the early 1990s. Vince McMahon had decided to start the equivalent of a World Wrestling Federation for bodybuilding and my father had agreed to take part and return to competition. Later, Joe Weider encouraged my father to come back to compete in Mr. Olympia, which he had never won, and then in the Masters Olympia. Dad was the youngest person to win Mr. Universe, which he had done twice, and had won a huge number of prizes and awards in his youth, but had never won Mr. Olympia.

He had been acting and doing personal appearances for over ten years at this point, so this was going to be a major change for our family. My parents knew this and sat us down for a family meeting when they decided my father would begin competing again. I remember sensing my dad was excited but my mom was nervous. While I understood something was changing, I didn't really get what this would mean for our family. It became clear soon enough.

Our family became a kind of business overnight, a business devoted to Lou Ferrigno's meals, diets, and needs. My mother worked from home, managing my father's career, and my dad began working out at the gym two times a day, for several hours at a time during each visit. He was counting every calorie and gram of protein he consumed. We began traveling, as a family, when he competed. My father always worked very hard and is 80% hard of hearing; this combination of factors has probably affected our relationship, which is now a good one, from the beginning.

While I never felt like I was Daddy's little girl, exactly, he was also fairly present when I was young — but as he began to intensely diet, work out, travel, and compete, our father-daughter bonding time became very rare. I told myself my father's new devotion to bodybuilding made him busy, but I understand now that I felt abandoned and was sad and angry about it.

Despite my parents' consciousness about our family changes, I also thought my feelings, and any role I was playing in this scenario, were my secret.

My mother was incredibly reassuring. My dad did the best he could and was always a loving father, but he was very focused on his goals and had to devote his time and energy in that direction. In addition to the changes in our family dynamics, my dad was also physically transforming before my eyes. He went from 240 pounds to 325 pounds and dropped down to 2% body fat.

As these changes continued, it became quite clear to me that his new profession was bullshit, and I felt resentful about the time it took away from our relationship. All the negative feelings I was having were coinciding, of course, with my beginning to age into adolescence. I began to resist anything that had to do with his new career. My parents, especially my mother, tried hard to keep some semblance of normalcy in the house — but the reality was we were not living in a normal situation. After I watched my dad put so much care into dieting and exercise, I rebelled against all of it. I blamed every healthy activity, every green vegetable, and every diet plan for taking my dad away from me.

I cursed the ground kale grew on, wanted to punch all low-fat foods in the face, and stuck both my middle fingers up at any quinoa that dared to get near my plate.

At ten years old, I did not understand my father was only following his passion and creating a better life for us. I also did not appreciate the difficulty of the challenge he had set for himself by deciding to return to competition at the age of 42. At the time, all I felt was that, somehow, his absence was my fault. I was hungry for my father's attention. Instead of knowing how to talk about the abandonment I felt, I replaced it. I filled the void I had with food. And it wasn't kale. I loved food but simultaneously feared it. I used food as comfort and as a weapon to take back some of the control I felt I was losing in the dynamic of my family.

Unlike my dad, I was fixated on enjoying everything that went into my mouth. My father is the most dedicated and determined man I have ever known. He leads by example in teaching the lesson of putting every ounce of your energy into your passion. In a strange way, this model worked against me as I used the focus and intensity I had been taught to eat anything and everything I wanted. If that meant I had to lie to get what I thought I wanted, I would. I began to lie about everything in order to fill my void.

Does any of this sound familiar to you? Our stories are individual, of course, but the shame of feeling out of control around our bodies, and the behaviors we develop to contain the feelings, come up over and over again as I work with people who struggle with their weight.

When I tell you I understand and that you can interrupt these patterns, whatever the specific details of your situation, it is not an empty promise.

To make the necessary changes, you must be willing to educate yourself and commit to this journey, which is not a quick weight loss scheme but a way of transforming your body as a part of living better. You will probably find you need to renew this commitment as you make progress, and sometimes you will take two steps forward and then one back. It's important to know this may happen and that you can keep going.

I was determined to keep building my comfort fort of food under my bed. It was an ultimate form of control for me. Some people become bulimic or anorexic to win back a sense of control with food by not eating it, or purging their bodies of what they consumed; I did just the opposite.

As much as I hated calories, and was aware of their importance in my father's life, I didn't really understand how they differ according to the nutrients they contain or why it wasn't good for me to constantly have them.

All I knew was I felt better, once I started consuming as many as I could. But the mirror and the outside world, especially the kids at school, continued to tell me otherwise. I was given a very hard time at school and, honestly, I was so unhappy that I was undoubtedly not offering up the most likable version of myself, which probably made things worse.

When kids and adults began to ridicule me is when my parents and I really started to take notice. I was starting to avoid mean students by hiding in the bathroom or cutting class altogether. My grades started to suffer and my parents decided I should start at a new school. The transfer resulted in my needing to repeat the fourth grade, and now I was going to be that much bigger, relative to my classmates.

Another turning point I remember from this year was that I was looking for an outfit for a special occasion and wound up finding something acceptable in a Lane Bryant. Lane Bryant stores, if you are not familiar, specialize in women's clothing in sizes 14-28. I applaud them for being early to the game of trying to offer fashionable options for larger women and helping people of whatever size feel good about how they look. As a fourth grader, however, needing to shop at a store for plus sized women made me different from my peers.

My father took me to see a nutritionist at his gym for the first time in this year. Her name was Kathy and she put me on a very sane eating plan that had an adequate number of calories balanced between protein, fats, and carbohydrates. We'll talk more about these issues later in this book. She educated me about nutrition; I was interested in what she had to offer, and was compliant with her slow and steady plan.

Following the nutritionist's strategies and learning about these issues also turned out to be a healthy way

of bonding with my dad.

Then I got very sick with the flu. My illness, combined with the lower number of calories I was eating and the beginnings of a growth spurt, caused me to lose 25 pounds quite quickly and I started feeling pretty good about how I looked. Due to the extraneous factors contributing to rapid weight loss, and the fact that I had changed my eating habits but not really addressed the core issues leading to my unhealthy habits in the first place, I didn't stick with the plan.

By sixth grade, while I wasn't as heavy as I had been in the past, I gained back some of my weight and was wearing size 10 or 12 clothes. Even though I looked more "normal" for my height I had not fundamentally resolved my issues with food or my body.

Still, I had experienced a taste of what it was like to feel excited when I looked in the mirror. I asked to consult with Kathy for a second time during seventh grade. This time, I really committed myself to a healthy eating and exercise plan and became very participatory in cooking my own food. I started weighing my food during this period and became obsessive about it. I also developed more enthusiasm about working out and finding ways to exercise that I enjoyed.

The treadmill really worked for me and I became obsessive about using that as well.

While I was getting physically healthier, my mental state related to food and body issues was transforming, but not necessarily in a positive way. My intensity about exercise caused me to experience some injuries that interfered with my progress, including a torn ACL.

My weight stayed fairly stable through the rest of high school, fluctuating maybe 15 pounds at various times. Although my weight was normal, I still felt self-conscious and unworthy, like I was the kind of girl who people thought of as fun, but not beautiful, or the best friend who would never get the guy. Then I went to college, which I loved, but doubled down on the clichéd "freshman fifteen" and gained thirty pounds. It was relative: I was now 5'8" and wearing a size 14, and while I had been bigger in the past, this still felt thick for me and it didn't feel great.

Then I went backpacking in Europe that summer with a girlfriend and the weight dropped off. It's funny, because hiking isn't my favorite thing to do, but I loved walking and sightseeing that summer, and lost 25 pounds in just a few weeks. I think I was very motivated by seeing some place new every day and discovering Switzerland, Italy, and Germany on foot. We'll discuss the importance of finding forms of exercise that inspire you later in the book, and while I do believe you need to chase the exercise you love for as long as the feeling lasts, it's important to understand the ways you like to move will also change in unexpected ways.

The other change I made over the summer was that I was instinctively creating a great balance between eating and moving. I was eating five or six small meals or snacks as I went everywhere rather than three meals a day, which is a fantastic way to stoke your metabolism.

I returned home in the summer of 2001 feeling like a 20-year-old badass and a small size 6. I was not skinny, but very fit and muscular, and got tremendous positive feedback from friends. Eventually, I found people were constantly asking me for advice on getting fit. I was living on my own in New York and felt responsible, successful, and excited about exploring different kinds of work and figuring out my life path. I started going to the gym again and using weights and then the treadmill for my main cardio workout, which is still one of my favorite ways to exercise. It was during this optimistic period that I got certified as a personal trainer.

At some point, one of my clients had a sister who lived in Austin, Texas and needed a house sitter while she was traveling. I fairly spontaneously decided it was time for a change and that it might be cool to spend some time in a new place. I moved into this magnificent house in Austin, and got a job working for a health-related nonprofit, where I was working on a smoking cessation initiative. I did not know many people in Austin, but found several who were thrilled to meet me and party in my borrowed, beautiful, 9,000-square-foot house. While I was working during the day, and excited about the potential in my job, I was also lonely and a bit unmoored.

This time, in addition to treating my loneliness and fear with food, I added alcohol to the mix as well. Instead of acknowledging I felt lost and scared, I developed a little swagger.

I was drinking and eating a lot with my new "friends" and staying up late. I kept both my fear and my drinking a secret from my colleagues. I couldn't keep my weight gain a secret — I gained 30 pounds in Austin and was back in size 36 jeans. No one knew me, though, so I thought I could be someone new, and imagined I couldn't embarrass anyone in my family. Again, my weight gain was not as disproportionate as when I was a kid, but I was bigger than I had been in a long time. Actually, when I think about this time, I remember I was mostly wearing leggings or anything with an elastic waist, as a little form of denial about my weight gain. I even started trying to mask my weight gain by wearing fake eyelashes, hair extensions and long acrylic nails.

My family saw me for the first time when I was about six months into this new phase. We were all meeting up in Ohio, where my father was being presented with a lifetime achievement award at the Arnold Schwarzenegger Classic. They took one look at my bloated face, blonde highlights, dramatic nails, and false eyelashes and started laughing. While I admitted I was eating too much this time, I didn't let anyone know how reckless I was becoming with alcohol. I decided to start my own nonprofit organization devoted to addressing childhood obesity, which I worked on during my off hours in Austin.

Because I was an obese kid, I thought I had something unique to offer families struggling with this issue. I also thought helping others and getting back to basics in this area could be healing for me. I knew I was spinning out of control, but I also knew I had confronted these issues successfully before. I thought this would be a way to touch base with myself again and deal with my substance and food abuse issues.

My non-profit in Austin was small and very local, but I was working directly with some groups and individual families on my own time, to guide them about exercise and food choices, usually because at least one child in the family had gained an unhealthy amount of weight. I remember sitting in the kitchen of an immigrant family with an obese child. I was talking to them about the economics of frozen vegetables, the importance of eating together as a family, and how much it would help if all their family members made the same dietary changes so their child would not feel singled out or punished. They were kind and well-meaning people but they didn't speak English well. They were having difficulty understanding why their own behavior was so important, and looked at me with genuine bewilderment. I remember taking a moment to try to figure out how to communicate more clearly with this family, and having this physical sensation of dread. I thought about what I must look like to these people, with my body reflecting months of secret late night eating and drinking. I knew I was preaching a message I wasn't committed to practicing. I felt like a fraud. Being able to have clarity about those feelings helped me create my own reset, and I thought, "game on."

My moment of clarity, of admitting I felt like a fraud and understanding I had been lying to myself, made me want to change. Sitting with those feelings and confronting the truth led me to find my purpose again and ultimately led me to create Ferrigno FIT and the Incredibly FIT program. I left Austin within the month and moved back home with my family in Santa Monica in order to get structure back into my life, and to save money. I recommitted to working out and started to develop the idea for Incredibly FIT. I also stopped drinking. While I was not an alcoholic, I did attend AA and Alanon meetings during this period.

Understanding the similarities between food and alcohol addiction made me see the need for a holistic fitness program that went deeper than just a diet or exercise plan and influenced how I ultimately developed Incredibly FIT.

As my plan took shape, I started working with my father and my friend Marti to bring Ferrigno FIT to life. As I have learned so many times, one positive choice led to another. Working with my father has not only led to professional success and a company that we are proud of, but also strengthened our relationship and helped me deepen my understanding of him, as well as my own issues about food and body image.

Look — *The Reset Plan* is designed to help you lose weight, but it can also be a tool to help you achieve so much more. If you commit to addressing your secrets and lies, you can not only become happier and healthier than you are right now, you can locate your purpose and unleash your potential. These are dynamic steps and the advice in this book is designed around the understanding that we are constantly changing. When we pay close, honest attention to our bodies, our feelings, and our behaviors, we can recognize our changes, identify our needs, and take action to be the best versions of ourselves.

This is not going to be easy. You will not lose a pound a day for a month. You are not going on a diet. You will not have low energy or weird food restrictions or complicated regimens to follow. You do not need to tell everyone your darkest fears.

You *do* need to take a hard look at your life, set your own goals, and figure out what you are capable of achieving. You can start small, but you are going to commit to a way of eating, exercising, and living that will, at a minimum, improve your health and happiness. If you give this plan a little time, you will feel a change in your stamina and inspiration you can access to maximize your potential. This isn't magic. You are going to have to work really hard, but you owe it to yourself to try. You are worth it. Throughout this book, we are going to explore why you and I hold on to feelings from our past and transform them into harmful secrets of our own.

We are going to confront the "10 Basic Lies We Tell Ourselves" that hold us back from achieving our true potential, and establish the tools we can use to interrupt them every time they cross our minds. Then, we are going to reset.

I still find certain things challenging about managing my own health and weight. I have had to tell my friends I am skipping a weekly margarita night in order to go to a fitness class, or that I would rather go to the gym if I hadn't already met my workout goal for that day or week.

When I first started doing this, if my friends gave me a guilt trip about it, I would give in and skip the gym. What I began to notice was when I skipped the gym twice in one week, I would sit at the restaurant, mad as hell at myself for allowing my friends to talk me into being there. In addition to not having a good time, instead of leaving immediately or confronting my feelings, I did what I am good at: eating and drinking.

I would eat more than usual and wasn't even in good spirits because of the guilt I had for not living up to my word. We all succumb to peer pressure for understandable reasons: we want to be a good friend, we genuinely don't want to miss out on a fun plan, or perhaps have fear we might be talked about if we are absent. What we often forget is the primary relationship we need to honor is the one we have with ourselves. It sounds selfish but it is actually necessary to be a good partner, parent, and friend. I think of it in terms of the disaster scenarios they prepare you for when your airplane is about to take flight: you are always advised to put your oxygen mask on first before helping others. I decided to write this book because I could not find anything out there linking the idea of self-care and psychology back to being FIT in the way I think we need to understand these concepts.

You need to feed yourself emotionally as well as physically and it's an ongoing process.

This book is packed with tools and plans to help you get wherever it is you need or want to go. Throughout this journey I promise to be as real and honest as possible, and I hope you do the same. It's time to let go of failure and frustration, get real, face your feelings and live your truth. You are about to begin *The Reset Plan: Lose the Secrets, Lose the Excuses and Lose the Weight*.

EXCUSE #1:
I'VE TRIED EVERYTHING AND NOTHING WORKS

When clients say this to me, what they usually mean is "diets don't work." And that is true. Even when you put your all into a diet, you are destined to fail. The diet is in control from the start to the end date, and that's assuming you obey it during this period. But we each have one start date in life — our birthdays — and I am grateful I don't know my end date. I want to make sure I give every day my all, and that means I need to be operating with all my power.

Diets cause most people to become obsessive and leave us feeling deprived physically, emotionally, and spiritually. When I feel deprived, I get resentful and angry. When I am forbidden from having a few pieces of cheese and crackers while everyone else is munching away I feel like I am being punished even though I want to live a healthier life — believe me, no one wants to be around me while I am dieting. I may have lost pounds on various diets over the years, but I'm sure I came close to losing the company of friends during those times as well!

Here are some hallmarks of a fad diet:

- You have no plan to keep weight off for the long run
- You're only allowed limited categories of food
- You're promised weight loss from a certain part of your body
- You're guaranteed to lose a certain number of pounds in a certain number of days
- You're always hungry
- You're following a plan based on a single study
- You have a list of "good" and "bad" foods

Sound familiar? If you have been sprinting from diet to diet all your life and are sick of starting and stopping and failing just to start again, it's time to start jogging alongside me as we train to become marathon runners together in pursuit of a sustainable lifestyle. You haven't tried everything yet. You might have tried the wrong things, or maybe you have been giving up your power.

It's time to get the voice out of your head that keeps saying you need to be told what to do or you will never be successful.

So many people tell me they hate to diet, but at the same time are convinced they need the food restriction. I hear people say all the time, "This diet is good for me because it doesn't allow me to keep the food I like in my house. If I buy it, I'll eat it." And you know what? It's true. Once most people lose some weight and are off the diet, they return to their old habits of buying what they like and eating too much of those foods — it's not really surprising.

When the diet is over, people believe they can become themselves again, which often means rewarding or comforting with food, which they often believe they can handle successfully this time around, since they've successfully reached a diet goal. This time period of perceived success is often when the habit of binge eating begins again. If this sounds familiar to you, it's time to be the hero of your own life and take responsibility for your actions. You can no longer blame a diet for letting you down, because you are done with diets.

Failure is when you give up your power in life. We all get knocked down, but it's not real failure until you choose not to get back up. Here's the thing: it's easier to stay on your feet if you know what to look out for on the road ahead and understand why you kept falling to begin with. Your road to optimal fitness as a part of your purposeful life is a long one, and it's dynamic; it will change as you change, and you need a fitness strategy to carry you through these changes.

If you need to lose weight, it's not just because you ate one bad meal — just like if you are depressed, it's not just because you had one bad day. Many people think that they can tolerate some deprivation in the short-term in order to get the benefits in the long-term, but it does not work that way with weight loss. Even if you experience some short-term success, you are very unlikely to sustain it.

According to a study reported by ABC News, 108 million people are on diets in the U.S.; dieters typically make 4-5 attempts per year.

85% of customers using weight loss products and services are female.

Since this is your personal journey, I don't know where you are right now or how long it will take you to reach your goals. Some of us have more to chisel down than others to get to our optimal emotional, physical, and spiritual places. What I do know is that I have worked for over a decade with hundreds of clients using the same strategies I am sharing with you in this book, and the principles I'm sharing work.

The clients who start with a positive attitude, an open mind, and on their own terms gave up their old ways of thinking tend to become healthier, happier, more fit, more optimistic, and more productive as they make progress. You are going to **Focus**, **Invest**, and **Take Action** to make yourself the priority for the rest of your life. You will never go back to dieting again. You will not be led by anyone or anything other than yourself. Acknowledge the past — all of it: the lessons, the blessings, and the pain — all that has led you to right here in this moment.

Your journey toward a new lifestyle can be a lonely one at first. You are going to have to accept that not everyone is going to understand or support you, which is tricky but common, and you should be prepared to deal with this hurdle. During the first six days, you are going to spend some time becoming self-aware about why you have tried different diets, trends, and fads; why they haven't worked; and whether there are people or things in your life undermining your efforts to be FIT. This task can seem daunting, but remember: none of this is new, and you are not alone.

If you're up for the challenge, keep reading. If you are ready, but scared, I am with you through this and promise to make this time in your life entertaining and stimulating. If you're not ready at this moment, be honest with yourself and put this book down until you are; it might be in an hour, a day, or even a month, but that's okay. If you don't take this journey on your terms and time, you'll just negate and resent what's happening, and even my methods won't work. I don't want to sound condescending, but it is important to have realistic expectations before you jump into the first six days.

THE FIRST SIX DAYS

Welcome to the first six days of *The Reset* of your life. As you follow your fitness journey, you should see changes each week, and we will upgrade your program every seventh day. Your program will renew until you reach your goal, wherever you set it, and can also be used to maintain your optimal level of fitness indefinitely. Don't get overwhelmed; this week is all about preparation. Focus on one day at a time.

I am not making you do 2 hours of cardio a day and starving you now or ever. I want to make it clear from the beginning, the first 6 days is about reflecting and self-monitoring. It is about increasing your awareness with how active you are daily and your food intake. As much as I do encourage you to get moving, the goal is to check in mostly with you. This is a HUGE part of this reset.

Setting Goals

One of the most fascinating parts of my job is helping clients set goals and discover what motivates them to take care of themselves, because everyone is so different. You will need to determine your own goals this week and decide how you want to measure your progress. Measuring progress is no longer going to be dictated by the scale.

Instead, I encourage you to begin measuring your progress through inches lost, improved strength, endurance, appearance, energy, and mood, among other things.

Remember — the only person you need to compare yourself with is you. You should only be competing with yourself, striving to be better than you are today. First, you have to take a good hard look at where you are today. You can weigh yourself now, but please know you will put the scale away during this journey. I despise home scales and the obsessive head games they make so many of us play. Go ahead and record your starting weight — but then take time to review my diagram about how to measure your body to track your weight loss in other ways (see The *Reset Plan* Workbook at the end of this book). This will be the most accurate way to get results with the least amount of anxiety.

During this program, you will track and record your body measurements every seventh day. For the body measurements, you are going to measure your height-to-waist ratio as well as waist-to-hip ratio. You will measure your height and weight with a measuring tape. Your waist size should be less than half of your height. For example, if you are 5'2" tall (62 inches) the circumference of your waist should be less than 31 inches.

To get your hip-to-waist measurement you will measure each and then divide your hip measurement with your waist measurement. Compare your findings with the chart (see workbook) and keep track in your journal so you can watch these numbers change. Body measurements are a more accurate gauge of fitness and change than measuring your BMI.

If you have been on diets before, you're probably familiar with BMI. In case you are not, BMI stands for Body Mass Index and is supposed to be a measurement of your body composition based on a calculation of your weight and height. There are many online calculators to help you calculate yours, but I don't think the BMI is useful because it does not differentiate between the amount of bone, muscle, and fat in your weight, which all make a big difference.

Bone is denser than muscle, and twice as dense as fat, so a person with strong bones, good muscle tone, and low fat will have a high BMI; athletes and fit, health-conscious celebrities who work out a lot tend to find themselves classified as overweight or even obese. The BMI was created in the 19th century by a mathematician, not a doctor, and is a quick and easy way to measure the degree of obesity of the general population, but it does not have the sensitivity and accuracy that body measurements will provide for your journey.

Another way to monitor yourself as you go along is with your clothes. Grab a pair of pants, shorts, or a skirt you want to wear but is tight on you. Set them out where you can see them easily. Try them on whenever you are having a self-sabotaging moment. Their fit will not lie.

In order to monitor and appreciate the improvements you are about to make, you need to be clear about your starting point. Taking body measurements is something you can do yourself. Before I take on a client, I ask them to consult a physician. I do this for them, not me. You have to know yourself inside out to set your goals appropriately and get your best results. A basic physical is a must and blood work is encouraged, even though I'm sure some of you get as anxious as I do when it comes to giving blood. *Please do it.*

Your blood chemistry will help you focus on what your body needs. It will save you time, discouragement, and anxiety: most of my clients get the motivation they need once they see their blood work. It's also important for you to have a complete physical so old or new injuries can be evaluated. You will need to record the results of your exam so we will review that later in the chapter.

This may sound unconventional, but I want you to set a non-physical goal for this week as well. Choose a project in your house, car, or office that has been sitting on your to-do list for a while and make a commitment to execute it during the next six days. You can go ahead and identify additional tasks you might complete during the coming weeks and rank them in importance or the order in which it might make sense to complete them based on your schedule.

This week, mine would be my hall closet. It's my go-to place to throw junk into right before company comes over. I always promise myself I will organize the space, but I seem to always have an excuse about having no time to do it. I kept ignoring this project because I felt no one would see all the junk in there so I could put it off as long as I wanted. And you know what? It was the damndest thing: I noticed I felt guilty every time I walked by that closet and began to recognize it becoming a secret mental burden.

We all carry these nagging feelings around regarding unfinished business.

During this program, you will start and finish ten projects of this type, one each week. This is not an extra: your emotional well-being is connected to your physical well-being, and improving one will enhance the other. As you complete these tasks, you will be shedding mental burdens along with extra physical weight and will experience an increase in emotional energy along with physical strength. If it's broken, doesn't work, or is missing parts, throw it out. If you don't use it, give it away. If it's unfinished, make the time in the next eight weeks to complete it or remove it from your list.

FOCUS: Assess your physical and mental health. Envision your best self.

INVEST: Make a doctor's appointment. Locate or purchase a tape measure and take some key body measurements.

SELFIE "BEFORE" SHOTS: Take front, right, and left — and back, if possible.

TAKE ACTION: Put your scale away. Check a nagging project off your to-do list.

Understanding Yourself

You are going to spend this week auditing your food, your feelings, your exercise, and the people around you. You need a journal to record your observations. If you don't have something around the house you want to use, you can find inexpensive ones at any stationery, office supply, or super-store. Wherever you buy it, I want you to find a journal with a cover you find inspirational.

You can also create something personal by cutting and pasting an image or quotation onto an ordinary notebook. It's worth spending a few minutes on this project. Your journal is going to be your passport to your new adventures and will become a priceless compass to remind you why you started, and will keep you headed in the right direction on the days you might be tempted to throw in the towel.

Make sure your journal cover resonates with the way you envision your final passport page. Mine says "Be Your Own Hero."

Leave the first five pages of your journal blank for now. You will eventually use these to record the numbers from your blood work and physical, along with any notes or suggestions from your doctor. These are your starting points and your benchmarks. I know it can take time to book an appointment, but ideally you will have some results during the first weeks of this process.

Make three columns on the sixth page of your journal and label them: LUST, LOVE, and INDIFFERENT. Write down ten foods under each column that makes you feel the corresponding emotion. As your relationship with food changes in the coming weeks, it's going to be interesting to watch.

Leave the third and fourth pages open to track your biweekly measurements. Take them this week and then again every other week on your upgrade day. Many people find tracking these measurements is more telling and more satisfying than tracking your overall weight on the scale.

There may be weeks when you are losing inches but not pounds, and as you become more fit and lean, measuring will help you pay attention to how your body is changing.

During the next six days, I want you to write down what and when you eat and how you are feeling when you eat it. If this sounds intimidating, don't worry: this level of detail won't be required forever, although some of you may find you enjoy it and want to continue, and that's great! Right now, just commit to keeping a journal of your food and feelings each day for the next six days. Writing down your food and feelings will help you become mindful about your habits. It will also be helpful if you record when you feel anxious about anything and how you deal with it, whether or not it has anything to do with food.

Try not to judge yourself while noting your observations. I always say be careful about the way you talk about yourself, because you're listening. There is no reason to ever be ashamed about your feelings; they are yours to have, and will continue to change. As you make an effort to be mindful and self-aware, the feelings or behaviors that are discouraging or embarrassing will change. Be proud; you are taking the first step of a critical journey. Here is an honest example of a journal entry of mine:

DAY 4

Shanna Victoria Ferrigno

It's 9:06pm, I'm exhausted, & have a really busy day tomorrow. I just got back from visiting my parents & childhood home. Being introspective this week, I realized the first thing I do at their house is head straight for the fridge. Hungry or not I always seem to set the tone around food. That house brings out emotional feelings for me and their fridge is, and always has been, a sanctuary of sorts for me. I stood in front of the half opened door and checked in with myself. I wasn't hungry, I just had a tough day. I grabbed the water bottle, closed the fridge & went into the living room to visit with my parents. NIGHT!

Being proud does not mean you have to talk about it with anyone right now. In fact, I don't encourage you telling a lot of people about your new lifestyle during this week. This is *your* time to observe your feelings, your routines, the people that support you, the way you speak to yourself, how you react to anxiety, anger, and identifying what frightens you. You will actually be doing more effective detective work if you keep your project to yourself for a few days.

Writing in a focused journal like this one comes more naturally to some people than others. If you need some inspiration and find yourself craving something, try considering these questions:

- Am I hungry?
- Why am I hungry?
- How much water have I had?
- Is my environment affecting my hunger? If I eat this, how will I feel afterwards?

If you just ate, feel free to record how you feel along with what you ate:

- Where and when did I eat?
- Did I enjoy my food?
- Was I distracted while I was eating?
- How do I feel? Satisfied? Energized?
- Still hungry?
- Bloated? Tired? Something else?
- Were my feeling different before, during, and after I ate?

You do not have to answer each question every time you write. The purpose of this exercise is to notice your patterns and become mindful of your relationship with food. I'd rather see you make a quick note than nothing at all if you are pressed for time because you'll still be able to identify patterns over the next six days if that's all you have.

If you take the time to explore your feelings more deeply, you'll get more out of this exercise. Whether you write for two minutes or twenty, it's important to record the date, time and feeling.

JOURNAL SUGGESTIONS/SAMPLE PAGES:

Plan Ahead

You cannot be successful with anything in life without attention and planning. It's *vital* to understand your own time. You will make changes every six days during this program and the upgrade day will always be on the seventh day. This day will become your **"FITamentalist" Day**, during which you will prepare for the next phase. Make sure you have about three hours to give to yourself and this important project on your seventh day. You are going to:

- Grocery shop
- Upgrade your food choices
- Prep your meals

Don't plan the seventh day to fall on a day that is hectic for you. If Sunday is the best day to prep your meals, organize your program to have the seventh day fall on a Sunday. If Wednesday is a better day for you, then plan to prep your meals on that day. The seventh day will be a day of physical rest and mental gain. Take a look at your calendar and figure out a plan you can stick to (more or less) to give this project the attention it deserves.

FOCUS: Become mindful of your eating habits and your routines. Notice your feelings and the way you talk to yourself.

INVEST: Buy or make a journal.

TAKE ACTION: Record your food and feelings this week. Plan some food prep time.

Inspire Yourself – Create a Mantra

You need to create a self-talk dialogue and a personal mantra.

This is something you will say to yourself every morning. It should inspire you to stay on track and remind you you're worth it, even when you don't feel like it.

I am *not* and have never been a morning person. Even as a kid, I always woke up grouchy. When I was young, I was convinced I was allergic to mornings and, as an adult, I used the excuse of "I *need* my coffee before I can function." I had convinced myself I "needed" the caffeine and felt so addicted that if I ran out of coffee, it could ruin my day.

Three years ago, one of my closest friends experienced a brain aneurysm and died suddenly. His death made me feel shameful about my morning tantrums. A circumstance, another person, or a situation can trigger shame in you, but so can failure to meet your own ideals or standards, especially when it comes to weight loss.

Shame can lead you to feel as though your whole self is bad or flawed, and can make you want to hide or withdraw from others. Shame actually lurks behind addictions in order to mask its impact. In fact, shame is often confused with guilt, something you might be willing to talk to others about, but when it comes to shame, that is often not the case.

Regardless of the trigger, when shame is experienced, your sense of self-esteem can go right out the window. It can be overwhelming, destructive, and devastating. You might feel anger, envy, anxiety, and even rage, not to mention depression or loneliness. A feeling of emptiness inside you can result from shame, and become a dangerous emotion because it can color how you view yourself. Shame can affect your self-esteem in a negative way. But you *can* recover from experiencing shame.

For example, instead of holding onto shame and guilt, I feel lucky enough to wake up and see each morning. I made the decision to change my thinking through my actions and created a self-talk dialogue and mantra. My morning dialogue is, "I am grateful to open my eyes to this new day. I am thankful that I have the strength and health to be able to work out today." Your self-talk dialogue should be something for which you are grateful and thankful at the moment.

Your **Personal Mantra** should be a positive statement you say to yourself for the purpose of encouraging yourself. The mantra could be your favorite quote, proverb, spiritual truth, or religious saying which motivates and inspires you to be your best self. Listen to the way you speak to and about yourself. If you can't say something nice about yourself, you're going to have to *practice*. Your mantra must be affirmative. For example: "I am not strong enough yet" will not help you — but "I am strong and getting stronger every day" works.

I have had many mantras over the years and change them up according to what inspiration I need at the moment. Right now, mine is "Life isn't about finding yourself — it's about creating yourself."

Not everything you do in your life will be done perfectly, but that's life and what being human is all about. I made my choices, and when I decided to own my actions, and their consequences, I began to learn from them instead of feeling embarrassed or stuck. I am recognizing those choices helped create the woman I am today.

FOCUS: Assess what motivates and inspires you.

INVEST: Create a personal mantra and a self-talk dialogue. Write them down in your journal.

TAKE ACTION: Say your mantra and dialogue each morning this week.

MAKING CHANGES: EATING AND DRINKING

The next six days are not about making drastic food changes; they are about evaluating where you are so you can figure out how to make effective change going forward. The focus of the next six days should be on preparing to upgrade your choices. However, there are three diet-related things I would like you to do this week, and they may be a challenge for some of you:

Eat Breakfast — I know, I know, some of you aren't hungry in the morning and don't want to waste the calories if you're not hungry. I've heard it all before and am here to tell you your metabolism will benefit by you eating a little something within an hour of waking up. I'm not telling you what you have to eat this week — we'll get into that next week — but eating breakfast is a *must* on this program and I'd like you to get into the habit.

Drink Water — Before you eat breakfast each morning, I want you to drink a pint-size or beer-size glass of water with lemon. This will hydrate you, give you a dose of Vitamin C, boost your immune system, and, for many, have metabolic benefits. When you are hydrated, any fine lines and wrinkles you may have will be less obvious, which allows you to look and feel better as well. Do not limit yourself to this one glass of lemon water if you like it! You benefit from being hydrated throughout the day and one way to monitor this is by noticing that your urine is pale yellow and clear. If it's not, your body is telling you you're dehydrated. Another tip is to take a gallon of water (8 pints) and mark the water jug with a time frame of every two hours. It is a great way to remind you to drink and shows you how much you are drinking.

Cut Out The Booze — If you are anything like me, you may gasp at this to-do and would want to know why wine is being taken away from you — especially if you are Italian, like me. Don't get all worked up yet. Though excluding alcohol is encouraged, it's only mandatory these first six days. Just like I want you to check in with your food habits, I want you to do the same with alcohol. Your mind needs to be clear morning, noon, and night. In the morning, you can blame being hungover for your mood. In the afternoon, you might crave something greasy because of your hangover. At night when you have that habitual alcoholic beverage, it will alter your food choices.

We are not blaming hangovers and diets anymore. They both set you back and give you a symptom to blame for your bad habits.

Take alcohol out of your diet altogether during the next six days. You will be able to add it back in your routine later on if you choose, but it's really better not to drink during these prep days. Alcohol is dehydrating, and alters the way your body digests nutrients and utilizes sugars. We also tend to eat more and be less mindful of our food choices when we drink. Even if you don't regularly drink to excess, this is worth trying. Alcohol can blur your mindset and I really want you to be clear during this week of evaluation. It's only six days.

FOCUS: Become mindful about when and what you eat.

INVEST: Experiment with a few basic changes this week.

TAKE ACTION: Drink water with lemon each morning. Eat breakfast within an hour of waking. Eliminate alcohol for the next six days.

MAKING CHANGES: MOVING

Again, the goal of the next six days is primarily to figure out where you are. You don't need to wait a week to start walking, though. Start keeping track of how much you walk. This may be information you want to add to your journal, although some people find it more effective to use their phones or some other electronic device to track this. Whatever works for you is fine, the point is to figure out your baseline and start to find ways to increase movement during your day. Little changes here really add up: try walking up the stairs at work when you take a bathroom break. If you have been sedentary, begin walking for 10 or 15 minutes a day, at any pace that feels comfortable.

Invest in a pedometer or app to track your steps and how much you are walking each day.

A general fitness goal is ten thousand (10k) steps a day. Researchers at Arizona State University have established baseline activity levels based on the number of steps taken each day. People who take fewer than 5,000 steps are considered to be sedentary or inactive. Those who take 5,000 to 7,499 steps daily have a low active lifestyle. Somewhat active people usually take 7,500 to 9,999 steps per day and people considered active take 10,000 or more steps every day.

It's okay if you find you're walking a lot less frequently to start; do not judge yourself. Walking a mile is generally equivalent to two thousand steps and most people's work and home lives are structured so that getting ten thousand steps, or five miles, in each day requires a bit of thoughtfulness. Try taking a walk in the morning or after dinner, even if it's just fifteen minutes. Try taking stairs instead of the elevator, or parking further away from your office than you normal. Don't worry about getting your steps in all at once or how fast you take them.

When I started tracking my steps, I was at about 4k per day and now am routinely FAR surpassing a daily 10k. I found that increasing my steps was a fun game for me – you may feel the same way. However many steps you take a day when you start tracking, try to begin adding anywhere from 250-400 additional steps each day with a goal of consistently taking 10k each day. We will be adding fitness components throughout this program to help you become stronger and leaner, but try to think of the walking as a basic way of promoting your own wellness.

Many of my clients find being conscious of their steps helps them be more conscious of their food choices as well.

Experiment with different ways of walking. Some of my clients find that walking alone is meditative and calming, and becomes a centering time in their day. If you don't feel this way, try to make a date to walk with a friend or family member and catch up during a walk instead of a coffee. If you are walking alone, try making a playlist of music that makes you want to move and helps pass the time.

Audiobooks and inspirational podcasts (*stay away from the food ones, please*) are also a great trick to keep you on the treadmill or pass the time on a hike. If you really like what you're listening to, it might even encourage you to go that extra mile. Try walking at different times of day to see when you have the most energy. Do not give up on walking and don't let it get stale... you are in this for the long haul. Take note of your miles in your journal and be sure to record how you feel when you reach that 10k milestone for the first time.

FOCUS: Assess the amount of exercise you get regularly.

INVEST: Consider purchasing a pedometer/app or using some other way of tracking your steps this week.

TAKE ACTION: Increase the number of steps you take each day — or, if you have been completely sedentary, start walking for 10-15 minutes each day.

Educating Yourself

Part of being conscious of your food choices requires educating yourself about your nutritional requirements and the contents of your food. I want you to understand the Healthy Plate and exchange list (see The *Reset Plan* Workbook); how closely do your current food choices match the recommendations? I have also listed four different caloric and lifestyle suggestions. Consider which suggestion might be a good fit for you as you prepare to step up your food game next week.

While I want you to hide your body weight scale, invest in a food scale if you feel you can. A food scale can make your life easier and keep you honest about portion sizes as you move forward with the plan. If you do not want one, there are some fun ways to identify portion sizes without a scale:

- Deck of cards or an iPhone 5 = 3 ounces of meat or poultry
- 1/2 baseball = 1/2 cup of fruit, rice, pasta, or ice cream
- Baseball = 1 cup of salad greens
- 4 dice = 1-1/2 ounces of cheese
- Tip of your first finger = 1 teaspoon of butter or margarine
- Ping pong ball = 2 tablespoons of peanut butter
- Fist = 1 cup of flaked cereal or oatmeal or a baked potato
- Compact disc or DVD = 1 pancake or tortilla

Look at the foods you have been eating this week. What are your true portion sizes? If they are a lot larger than the recommended ones, try a little experiment. If your normal portion size of rice, for example, is two baseballs, try eating a quarter of your normal portion (a half baseball is the recommended portion size) and then wait for at least twenty minutes before going back for the rest of your normal portion. How do you feel? Write it down!

If you would like to get a personalized meal plan or have questions answered by a professional dietitian, you can go to FerrignoFIT.com. Even if you're not ready for a personalized meal plan, you can also choose a sample meal plan to follow — Sample Plans are now in the workbook at the end of this book.

Finally, I'd like you to take a field trip this week to your grocery store. Think about the perimeter of your grocery store. The whole, healthy foods are all there, right out in the open: produce, eggs, and meat. The inside aisles hold most of the preservatives, artificial sweeteners and all around fake food crap. Relate to the grocery store like you would your secrets. You can't ignore the middle aisles, just like you can't ignore your secrets or shame, but you don't have to feed off of them. Knowledge is power.

When you look at labels on your staple items, ask yourself:

- What is the name and form of the food?
- Who is the manufacturer?
- What is the largest ingredient?
- What is the serving size?
- How many servings are in the container?
- Are there more than 5 ingredients?

Go through those middle aisles and identify all the preservatives and nutritional profiles on items you might normally choose. Do the same thing with foods you buy from the outside perimeters of the store. You will use the information you find to upgrade your ingredients and choices in the coming weeks. We will discuss the importance of nutrients, fiber and macros in the chapters ahead.

FOCUS: Educate yourself about optimal nutritional requirements and portion sizes.

INVEST: Consider purchasing a kitchen scale.

TAKE ACTION: Compare your food choices this week to the recommended ones. Take time in the grocery store this week to really examine the contents of your usual purchases.

Prepare Your Kitchen

You are going to rediscover your palate on this plan, which means you are probably going to be more involved in preparing your food than you used to be. Pay attention to your five senses. I promise, your tastes are going to change throughout these phases as you upgrade your diet. We are going to bring you back to the feeling of smelling, tasting, and enjoying different foods for the first time. We are not depriving ourselves, but reducing deprivation of taste and flavor many of us have developed through poor eating and yo-yo dieting. Our lives will be so much easier when our kitchens are in order and we have the proper tools for making quick, healthy meals.

Assess Your Equipment — You are going to be doing more cooking and food preparation in the coming weeks. Assess your kitchen equipment and make sure you have a working set of pots and pans, a scale for weighing your food, a good set of sharp knives, a blender, and Tupperware or other food storage containers. None of these items need to be fancy or expensive, and they are all worth investing in if you don't already have them. Consider investing in a grill, measuring spoons, salad spinner, spiralizer, a food cooler, and/or Tupperware or other food storage containers if you think they might help you.

Consider Small Plates — Consider downsizing some of your bowls, plates and utensils, particularly if you have a lot of the oversized or restaurant-sized dishes that have been fashionable in the last few years. Many people find it more satisfying to arrange and eat smaller portions from something about the size of a kid's dining set or salad/appetizer-sized plates. Don't worry — you don't have to buy a whole new dinner set. You can find inexpensive small plates from many sources (possibly at the same place you choose to buy your journal). HomeGoods has an excellent selection of fun, designer dishes at rock-bottom prices.

Like your journal, make sure your small plates have a design that is appealing and inspiring to you. I discourage black plates as well as plates with bright red and yellow together. Studies have shown those colors cause your appetite to increase; maybe this is why so many fast food restaurants are covered in yellow and red.

Clean Out Your Cabinets — Okay, on day six, it's time to clean up your kitchen cabinets. Ditch anything that has more than five ingredients on the label and/or any ingredient you can't pronounce. That's right: give it to a local food drive, your neighbor, throw it away or just get it out of your kitchen. Make sure you do not go to the grocery store and buy more of this crap. You will thank me later. Begin by looking for these ingredients:

- **Hydrogenated Oils (any kind)** – found in: most processed foods, breads, flavored yogurt, salad dressings, canned vegetables, cereals

- **Trans Fats** – found in: margarine, chips, crackers, baked goods, fast foods
- **Monosodium Glutamate (MSG)** – found in: Chinese food, many snacks, chips, cookies, seasonings, name-brand soup products, frozen dinners and lunch meats
- **Sodium Sulfite** – found in wine and dried fruit
- **Sodium Nitrate** – flavoring in bacon, ham, hot dogs, luncheon meats and other processed meats
- **High Fructose Corn Syrup**
- **BHA and BHT** – found in: cereals, chewing gum, potato chips and vegetable oils
- **All Artificial Sweeteners** (Stevia, Splenda, Aspartame)
- **Anything with food coloring, such as Blue #1 and Blue #2** – found in candy, cereal, soft drinks, sports drinks
- **Red #40** – found in: fruit cocktail, cherry pie mix, ice cream, candy and bakery products
- **Yellow #6** – found in American cheese, macaroni and cheese, candy, carbonated beverages, lemonade, etc.
- **Any label that says "artificial" or "food product"**

If you have items with these ingredients, please just throw them out and don't look back. These guidelines should have caused you to effectively eliminate:

- Most chocolate or candy
- Potato or corn chips
- Soft drinks
- Low fat or fat free snack items
- Instant anything

I bet we just made a lot of space in your kitchen. That's great because now there should be room to add a lot of fresh and frozen, non-starchy vegetables (refer to food list)

You also need to look at the food remaining in your cabinet and read labels the way you did in the grocery store. Take some time to identify what I like to call the "White Zombies" that drag your energy down in your food: salt, sugar, and enriched flour. I am not telling you to eliminate products containing these ingredients right now; I just want you to notice when these ingredients are present in your food and in what quantities. Remember, this week is all about assessment, and you are probably getting more salt, sugar, and enriched flour than you think you are. Read the labels carefully and keep in mind the multiple ways products might list these ingredients on the label.

FOCUS: Prepare to start seriously improving your diet, the quality of your meals and how they're prepared.

INVEST: Consider purchasing or borrowing any kitchen equipment that might facilitate your preparation of healthy meals.

TAKE ACTION: Clean out your kitchen cabinets. Round up a few small plates. Buy more vegetables. Get excited to cook.

DAY SEVEN: YOUR FIRST *FITA*MENTALIST DAY

Review your journal and think about what you have observed this week about your relationship to food, movement, and your environment.

Questions To Consider:

- Did you notice patterns in the times of day or night when you made poor food choices?
- Are there any foods or meals that seem hard for you to "control" yourself around?
- How did you feel about the nutritional profile of the foods that are part of your regular grocery list?
- Can you identify factors in your routines that made it easier or harder to fit in some extra movement?
- How do you feel this week after increasing your movement? Were you sore? Tired? Energized? Happier?

- Do the people you spend your day with follow healthy lifestyle habits like exercising, and watching what they eat?
- Does your partner follow a healthy lifestyle?
- If you go out and eat more than once a week, do the people you eat with order healthy items?
- If you wanted to be active and go for a hike or the gym, how easy is it to find someone to go with you?
- Do the people you live with bring home foods that could contribute to your weight gain?
- When you look in the mirror are you upset, humiliated, or frustrated by what you see?
- When you're tired or feeling run-down do you blame it on getting older or your stressful environment?

You are taking action to improve your health and your life. If your environment is not supportive, it may need a makeover because your social group will be an important variable in your success. I am not saying everyone in your family must undertake the same journey, although it would be helpful, but it is *vital* you have a community that is supportive as you seek to break harmful habits. If you don't already have one, you'll need to make it a priority to start seeking one out this week. Fortunately, there are a lot of great resources online (including groups on our FerrignoFIT.com website).

MOVEMENT: THE UPGRADE

Today you are going to take a physical assessment test. This will be the only activity I will ask you to do on your upgrade day. It is important to do this assessment at least biweekly. It's great motivation and a better way to see how much more fit you are becoming as opposed to how much "thinner" you are on an unreliable scale. Five of the six tests will take only a few minutes each, and the entire project should take you less than an hour to complete — maybe considerably less time, depending on how comfortable you are with the movements this first time.

Always stretch to warm up your muscles before your FIT test to prevent injury. It might be fun to grab a friend or partner on your upgrade day to keep you motivated and to help each other with the tests. Making an afternoon of meal prep and fitness assessment tests is my idea of a real happy hour! Here are the six assessments I want you to take today and then work to improve on during the next week:

Walk/Jog

I know you have been walking and starting to track your steps this week. Now, I'd like you to upgrade and pay attention to how fast you are walking or, if you are running, how fast you are moving. If you have been walking and generally sedentary before this week, choose a relatively flat one-mile walk and just time yourself while you walk that mile without stopping.

Your goal should be to walk one mile within 15 minutes. That is a brisk pace, do not worry if it took you a lot longer — just be aware that this week, you're going to start to walk a bit faster to try to reach your 15-minute goal. If you walked a mile in 15 minutes, no problem; if you have already been jogging, go ahead, keep going and track your time. Your goal should then be a 10-minute mile, and again, don't worry if it took you longer. This is a starting point. Everyone is at a different point in their physical fitness journey —some of you might start out at a fast pace while others may need some time to work up to a longer walking time and pace.

Flexibility Assessment Test

Now that you're warmed up, you can take the stretch test. Remove your shoes and grab a yardstick or a ruler. Sit on a flat surface near a step or a wall with both legs extended in front of your body. Point your toes up and place your feet slightly apart, with the soles of the feet against the base of the step. Place the ruler on the ground between your legs or on the top of the step. Place one hand on top of the other, and then reach slowly forward. At the point of your greatest reach, hold for a couple of seconds, and measure how far you have reached.

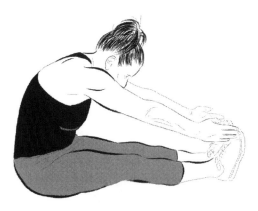

If you have trouble straightening your legs, get a friend to help by holding the knees down flush with the ground. Do this twice, and have you or your partner track your best distance. Don't worry if you are not able to stretch very far initially; you will improve in the weeks ahead. If your numbers are on the low end, don't get down on yourself. You will get there.

Posture Assessment Test

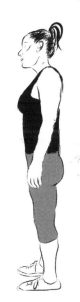

You are going to start weight training soon and I want you to make the most of it! It's so important to have good form to get optimal results from weight training and that requires good posture. If you need more motivation, the right posture will not only benefit you in the long run, but can instantly make you look five pounds thinner. Really! Not sure if your posture is on point? Look in the mirror or have your partner look at you. Your back should have an elongated S shape when viewed from the side. Follow these tips to make sure your body is in alignment:

Neck: Hold your head high and straight without tilting it forward or to the side. Your ears should be in line with the middle of your shoulders.

Shoulders: Pull your shoulder blades back and down to lift your breastbone.

Abdomen: Tuck your abdomen in, but be careful not to tilt your pelvis forward or backward.

Knees: Keep your knees slightly bent and shoulder-width apart.

Push-Up Assessment Test

Set a timer for one minute. Do as many push-ups as possible for that minute, or until you can no longer do anymore, if you can't make the whole minute. Count as you do them or have your partner count your total number of push-ups.

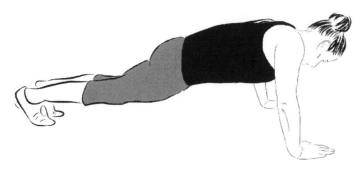

If you are at a medium to advanced level of fitness, feel free to use the standard "military style" pushup position with only the hands and the toes touching the floor in the starting position. I always tell women it's perfectly fine to use the "bent-knee" position. I am more concerned about your form than anything else. Bent-knee pushups are done by kneeling on the floor, placing your hands on either side of your chest and keeping your back straight. Lower your chest down towards the floor, always to the same level each time, either until your elbows are at right angles or your chest touches the ground.

Sit-Up Assessment Test

Set your timer for one minute again. If you have a partner, they can help count your sit-ups as well as help your feet stay on the ground. There are a few different ways of doing sit ups, depending on what feels most comfortable to you. Start by laying on a cushioned floor, mat or bench. Lay flat on the ground with bent knees, feet flat on the floor, and bent arms behind your head. Sit up, touch your knees with your elbows, then lie back on the floor. Repeat as quickly and often as possible for the next minute.

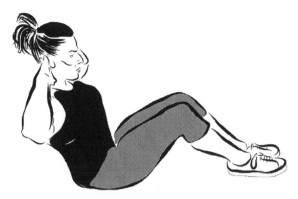

If this hurts your neck, try a modified version: Lay with your knees bent at approximately right angles, with your feet flat on the ground. Your hands should be resting on your thighs. Squeeze your stomach, push your back flat, and rise high enough for your hands to slide along your thighs to touch the tops of your knees. Don't pull with your neck or head, and keep your lower back on the floor by tightening your abdominal muscles, then return to the starting position. Once you have this motion down — and it's important to keep your lower back against the floor — repeat it as often and quickly as possible for the next minute.

Plank Assessment Test

If you can hold an abdominal plank position for at least two minutes, you're off to a good start. If you cannot, you're likely lacking in core strength, which is important for overall movement, stability and strength. A strong core will also help prevent back pain. Being unable to hold a plank for two minutes may also indicate that you're carrying too much weight, and would benefit from shedding a few pounds. Let's find out where you are.

Get in a modified push-up position with your elbows bent at 90-degree angles and both forearms resting on the floor. Position your elbows directly underneath your shoulders and look straight toward the floor. Your body should form a perfectly straight line from the crown of your head to your heels. Now just hold that position for as long as you can or until two minutes are up.

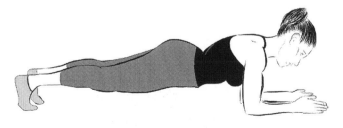

Some tips to consider while in plank position: One is to pull in your belly button. Then drive your chin down toward your toes while you're focused on squeezing your bellybutton in. Next, do a Kegel squeeze — more women than men might be familiar with this term: it means drawing your lower pelvic muscles up and holding them high and tight.

You know what's coming next, right? I want you to record the results of your fitness assessment in your journal. It's okay if the numbers seem low compared with the charts and guidelines provided. It's also normal for your results to be uneven, with one test or area much stronger or weaker than another. This is where you are, and you will only compete with yourself in the coming weeks as you get stronger.

CLIENT STORY: NANCY

"This is a decade overdue but I am ready to admit that I am done with all my excuses. They are literally killing me. I have not been intimate with a man for 12 years and haven't seen my vagina in at least a decade. It's the truth and I am ready to change or I am going to end up dead."

Well, damn. I instantly stood up and applauded Nancy. The woman had more strength in her truth than I believe she knew she even had. Nancy was "mad as hell and [she] wasn't going to take it anymore." Knowing this woman for all of 10 minutes, I knew any battle we would be taking on together would be a hell of a lot easier than her own battle she had been silently suffering from for over 2 decades.

Throughout her 46 years, Nancy had seen every dress size from 28 to 8. She had gone from being an overeater to an emotional eater and had hit her limit when she came to see me at 322lbs.

At 5'5", Nancy was tired of battling how she looked in the mirror daily. Every meal was a struggle. Nancy had been on every diet imaginable, and because nothing worked she didn't know who to trust or what method to use. Eat bread? Ditch bread? Don't eat after the moon sets in the evening? Eat breakfast only as the rooster crows? It was maddening, all the confusing advice she had digested over the years. Not to mention family and friends, all with "critical opinions," surrounded her — but no one ever offered to be active with her.

Nancy's mother was super-critical of everything Nancy did. At 5'3" and 110 pounds, Nancy's own mother was abused severely as a child and held her control with the food she had around her. Growing up, Nancy's lunches were measured and weighed. No sugar was ever allowed in the house and each lunch was never more than 600 calories. It was her mother's obsession that Nancy rebelled against.

"Shanna — I am so tired of starting and failing that I promised myself I would never diet again, and out of spite decided to live my life and eat whatever I wanted. I said this 100 pounds ago and am even more depressed trying to be happy that I am literally on the edge of suicide. I have so many people in my life that constantly criticize me, thinking that it will help me lose weight. If anything, it has caused me to not eat in public and hide what I eat when I am alone at home." Every time Nancy ate, the cycle was the same: bliss and happiness at first — but the more she ate and hid, the more numbness and disappointment crept in, masking all the joy. Like an addict, the disappointment of her actions always faded into shame.

"Visiting my mother, and the few days after, is what really triggers all the emotional eating. The moment I walk into the house, my mother will start commenting about how heavy I am. Trying to be 'helpful,' she will give me a pile of handouts or cutouts from magazines/ads she has collected about weight loss, detoxes, the newest weight loss tool/fad, and/or retreats that 'guarantee' long-lasting success."

For the last 5 years, Nancy never went out for the promotion she should have gotten at work because she had guilt and shame about the way she looked. In turn, she also felt like she didn't deserve it. She has a vision board of places around the world she wants to explore but hasn't made it realistic, because how is she going to go whitewater rafting at her weight, let alone budget for the extra seat she will need to fly comfortably for a 14-hour flight?

I started to work with Nancy twice a week. Sunday was usually when she would visit her mother. I would have her document her feelings about her visit and journal what she ate all week, specifically the day before and after her visits. After seeing the extreme difference of her portions and fast food visits, we decided to take a 30-day break visiting her mother to get her head adjusted to her new lifestyle. Each amount of time is different for people to help break the cycle friends and family members can evoke. Nancy believed 30 days of no visits would work for her.

We went moment-to-moment and day-by-day. Nancy would call her mother regularly but decided that 42 days was the right amount of time before visiting her mother again. She decided to change the habit of Sundays and go whenever she made the time. She realized she could not control her mother or her mother's actions; she only had the power to *RESET* her own.

Nancy lost 53 pounds and has consistently kept that weight off. Though progress is slow physically, after working with a therapist she started tackling demons she had no idea she had. She is growing mentally and that is what counts. Through our work, she learned how to eat healthy, how to eat one less scoop full of food each serving and ditch a ton of the processed foods. She is back in control of her life and the family and friends she surrounds herself with. She is confronting her shame, guilt and secrets daily. Her trip to Madrid is booked for April 2018. Regardless of the weight loss, Nancy is happy and accepting of herself now.

EXCUSE #2:
I DON'T TRUST MYSELF WITH FOOD

How you feel is just as important as how you look. Let's ditch the notion that you have no self-control when it comes to food. If you have to sneak to do it, lie to cover it up, or ignore the natural cravings of your body to avoid being seen or "judged," then you probably shouldn't be doing it. What would happen, for example, if we were to start thinking about food as less of a thing and more of a relationship? This is why I want you to come to terms with the idea that this week there will be no dining out. Have plans you can't miss? Start the day after — but this week you have to be devoted to staying consistent with your meal plan and being clear about your relationship to food.

"When you know better...you do better." – Maya Angelou

Diets through the decades have been all over the map with their suggestions. Drink this shake and lose inches on your waist. Eat this prepackaged meal and lose 10 pounds in 10 days. Whatever guarantee they are pitching it's vital to have the education behind it.

Walk into any grocery store. The outside perimeter of the market is filled with fresh fruit, vegetable, milk, eggs etc. When you go inside that perimeter is where you will find the cookies, chips and low fat dressings. Do you ever wonder how they can stay on the shelf for months and bagels for weeks on end and not expire?

It's the land of "inside the perimeter" where preservatives, sugar, sodium, and hydrogenated oils live.

Though it's a nice thought to only shop on the outside perimeters of the aisle, life happens. So, let's get real. Sometimes you have to go into the land of the lost nutrients to get to the Windex, water, or even toilet paper. Big companies are getting smarter with where they are placing items because they are onto the outside perimeter notion. I have a foolproof game that works for me when filling my cart up at the grocery store. I grab the item and ask myself these four questions:

- Is it unfamiliar?
- Can I pronounce all the ingredients?
- Are there more than 5 ingredients in the food item?
- Does it contain high fructose corn syrup?

All of these are crucial to identify when you are changing up your lifestyle. More often than not, if the item is or has ingredients that sound unfamiliar, you can't pronounce it, and has more than 5 ingredients, it's highly likely one of those ingredients is high fructose corn syrup. This is a *big* topic for me so I want to spend some time discussing what it is and why it even exists.

According to the United States Department of Agriculture, studies have shown the average person consumes half a pound of High Fructose Corn syrup a year. By 2010 people were consuming 43.5 pounds a year. I'm sure you have heard the media and TV experts warn you about High Fructose Corn Syrup and tell you how bad it is for your health? Do you know why?

High Fructose Corn Syrup (HFCS) originates from corn. It was discovered by the Japanese in the 1950s and made popular in the 1970s after President Richard Nixon elected Earl Butz as the Secretary of Agriculture. In 1971, our country was at war with Vietnam and President Nixon wasn't a crowd favorite. The cost of food was high and Nixon knew that unless he found a way to bring those costs down it could destroy his chance for a reelection.

Nixon brought in Earl Butz, an agricultural expert, who had good relationships with farmers and a plan of action. He ditched the motto of "supply and demand" and convinced the farmers to mass-produce corn. Corn would cut costs for companies and keep farmers in business because it could be used in everything. They fattened up the cows with it, they made oil from it, they put it in cereals — and the food science industry had officially begun. Food became big business. It was no longer about quality but about quantity.

Our country was becoming overfed and undernourished by ditching leaves for seeds.

Sweet corn is full of simple sugars. The starch from the corn is extracted and broken up into simple sugar (glucose) molecules that process into corn syrup. According to an article in the December 2008 issue of American Journal of Clinical Nutrition, corn syrup is 93% to 96% glucose. High Fructose Corn Syrup (HFCS) is produced when enzymes are added to the corn syrup. This converts (glucose) to another simple sugar called fructose. HFCS has 42 to 55 percent fructose that makes them similar to cane sugar. Take a look at the following terms:

Glucose — Derived from the Greek word *glukus*, meaning sweet. Glucose is a simple sugar that is an important energy source for living organisms and is found in many carbohydrates.

Fructose — Fructose is a simple sugar found naturally in fruits, vegetables, and honey. It gives them their sweet taste.

HFCS (High Fructose Corn Syrup) – Used in most products you see in your cookie aisle at your local grocery store. It makes everything sweeter than sugar because of how it is blended with other sweeteners. It was believed "innovative" because it keeps food moist for a longer period of time. It is less expensive than sugar and triples the shelf life.

Food prices went down, obesity went up, Nixon resigned from office, and Bentz was considered "revolutionary." Between 1970 and 1990, there was no food component Americans consumed more than HFCS. There was an outstanding 1,000% increase during these two decades; today it's the main sweetener in the U.S. for soft drinks.

Until the early 1970s, Americans believed fat and protein protected the body from overeating by allowing you to feel satisfied longer — the opposite of carbohydrates, which made you fat. In 1977, the U.S. Senate Select Committee on Nutrition and Human Needs, led by Senator George McGovern, came out with their first dietary guidelines and goals for the American people.

Heart disease was on the rise and they believed that by taking out saturated fat from your diet, it would be reduced. But in trying to address one problem with cutting back on fat, many experts I spoke with agree that the original dietary goals might have helped fuel other problems, like diabetes and obesity.

The U.S. Senate Select Committee consisted of manipulated politicians, not dietitians, leaving us all confused on our true dietary needs. Saturated fat needs to be limited, but all fat is not evil, and simple carbs are sugar, so not all carbs are good. But that message was lost in translation, and all Americans heard was "Fat is bad; carbs are good."

By the 1980s, "fat" had become "this greasy killer" and public enemy number one. Low-fat advertisers ran with the fact that because fat has nine calories per gram compared with four for protein and carbohydrates, carbohydrates were a healthier heart option. American breakfasts went from eggs, sausage and buttered toast to cereal with low-fat milk, unbuttered toast, and a glass of juice; hold the fat, but add the refined sugars.

Calorie – A calorie measures the energy in food and drinks we digest daily. You can't live a fulfilled life without energy. Energy comes in the form of calories, but not every calorie has the same amount of nutrients.

Eating 85 calories worth of blueberries (one cup) will process differently than 85 calories worth of Oreos.

Anything your ancestors would identify as food — fruits, vegetables, and protein — were no longer emphasized as nutritious. The '80s created the modernization of the Western Diet, a system that promoted nutrients, not food. They are not the same thing, but the misconception kept growing as our vocabulary did. The word "nutrient" is derived from macronutrients. Macronutrients consist of three things the body needs: carbohydrates, protein and fat. Each of these macronutrients consists of calories, but they all vary.

LET'S TALK ABOUT SUGAR

Most of the added sugar in the American diet comes from soft drinks, followed by sweetened fruit drinks, cake, candy and ready-to-eat cereals. Prepared foods like peanut butter, ketchup, and canned fruits and vegetables are also part of the mix. Any low-fat product where the fat has been reduced and replaced with sugar is another food type that you need to be aware may contain hidden sugars.

Food manufacturers add sugar to their products to not only make food sweeter, but also to improve and maintain the food's texture, color, and shelf life. When you're reading food labels, look for hidden sugars. Besides the word "sugar," they can be listed as the following:

- Corn sweetener
- Corn syrup
- High-fructose corn syrup
- Dextrose
- Fruit juice concentrates
- Lactose
- Maltose
- Malt syrup
- Molasses
- Cane juice

- Cane syrup
- Sucrose

Any ingredient ending in "-ose" is likely a form of sugar.

Lactose, found in milk, and fructose, found in fruits, occur naturally in these foods, but they also contain powerful antioxidants and nutrients our bodies need. It is the sugars and syrups added during process and preparation we need to be wary of. Plus, you need to be aware of any sugar you might add to a food or drink you make at home or when eating out.

In order to find those hidden sugars, look for the carbohydrate section on the food label and you should find the word "sugars" listed by weight. There is no difference between added sugars and naturally occurring sugars on the label. A good rule of thumb is:

If one or more of the first few ingredients on the list are forms of sugar, then it is likely the food is high in sugar. If the food product does not contain milk or fruit, then all the sugars have been added and you do not want to eat it.

You need to know sugar is why many people are overweight. According to the AHA, women should have no more than 100 calories of added sugar per day, which is is equal to 6 teaspoons. On average, most women are taking in 18 teaspoons a day.

1 teaspoon of sugar is equal to 4 grams of added sugar on labels

Too Much Sugar = Excess Carbs = A Fast Rise In Insulin Levels = Massive Fat Storage

Plus – sugar causes other health problems:

1. Sugar destroys the growth hormones to keep your body young and healthy.
2. Sugar damages eyesight, and increases the chances of getting osteoporosis.
3. Sugar can cause or contribute to eczema.

4. Sugar feeds cancer, spreading it through your body and devouring your healthy cells.

5. Sugar stimulates the production of insulin, which in turn makes your body more resistant to insulin and puts you at increased risk for diabetes.

6. Sugar jacks up your cholesterol levels, causing high blood pressure and heart disease.

7. Sugar beats down your immune system, fuels the growth of yeast inside your body, and throws your pH levels out of whack.

It does make you think twice about what you are putting into your body each day... all to get you going in the morning.

Do you love sugar? You are not alone. There are more than 600,000 food products that contain sugar and at least 80% have sugar added to them. These sugar-loaded foods literally become like addictive drugs. Doses of flour and sugar found in these foods alter our metabolism making us overweight and sick. Biologically, our bodies are addicted to sugar.

The American Journal of Clinical Nutrition has proven high-sugar foods are just as addictive as heroin and cocaine. They raise blood sugar quickly which triggers the pleasure centers of the brain, making you feel good and creating the urge for more of the same feeling. Foods that spike blood sugar are definitely addictive and they trigger a vicious cycle of cravings and hunger that set the stage for diabetes, heart disease, metabolic syndrome, and other chronic diseases.

When we were hunter-gatherers, we would binge on honey and berries when we could find them, which would help us store fat for hibernation during the winter months.

However, in today's world, we eat all winter long and not just high-sugar foods. There are millions of foods our ancestors would not recognize. We are literally ancient bodies living in a modern world and no one wants to be overweight or suffer from diseases. Unfortunately, willpower is not enough to overcome sugar cravings, especially if sugar and junk foods are in charge of your brain chemistry.

In a nutshell, high fructose corn syrup and other added sugars have stolen our hormones, metabolism, *and* our brain, creating this vicious circle of cravings and hunger. There is food, and there is junk food. Food created by nature does not come with an ingredient list, fake additives, preservatives, or barcodes.

The right foods send a message to our brain to shut down the cravings and hunger so we can burn body fat and feel energized. Processed, high-sugar foods send the complete opposite message, thereby creating the cravings for sugar.

HOW TO FIGHT SUGAR CRAVINGS

In order to fight sugar cravings, it is critical to choose unprocessed foods. In other words, if a food has more than five ingredients and a far-off expiration date, you do *not* want to eat it. Whenever you are tempted to eat a cookie or bag of chips, stop and ask yourself: What are you feeling? What do you need? Did you skip breakfast? Or eat an incomplete meal? Are you feeling emotional about a situation in your life? It is important to recognize our feelings and de-clutter our minds and bodies. Rewiring your brain can be done. Here are some smart strategies:

Eat REAL Whole Foods – This includes high-quality protein like fish, chicken, and eggs; good fats such as olive oil, nut butters, avocados; and whole food carbohydrates such as vegetables, legumes and nuts. We need some fat in our diet because it helps the body absorb certain nutrients. Fat is a source of energy as well as some vitamins (Vitamin A and D), and has essential fatty acids that the body can't produce on its own.

Eat Every Three Hours – This helps stabilize blood sugar levels throughout the day, preventing those sudden sugary cravings.

Think Protein And Fiber – Do this at every meal and snack. For example: eggs and vegetables, an apple with almond butter, or vegetables and hummus are all good choices. Meat is a good source of protein, vitamins, and minerals, including iron, zinc, and B vitamins.

Eliminate Refined Sugars – This includes fruit juices, soft drinks, and artificial sweeteners. These are like drugs that fuel addiction to sugar.

Reduce Stress – When you are stressed out, you are more likely to reach for something with sugar in it. Figure out what is stressing you out and address it by doing deep breathing, yoga, or meditation.

Walk It Off – Instead of reaching for that pint of ice cream, go for a walk. Exercise can eliminate or reduce cravings significantly as it raises the feel-good endorphin levels.

Know Your Food Sensitivities — You might be allergic to gluten, dairy, sugar, corn, peanuts or eggs. Are you eating something that is setting off a food sensitivity that could be causing your cravings for sugar?

Get Enough Sleep – A lack of sleep can increase cravings the next day. Shut down your computer at night at least one hour before bedtime.

Consider Supplements To Curb Cravings For Sugar – They include vitamin D3, omega-3 essential fatty acids, and chromium picolinate. When our bodies are lacking nutrients, it can set the stage for more cravings.

By supporting your body with good nutrition, you will be able to naturally let go of the cravings for sugar and junk food. You will notice an increase in energy and sense of well-being when you eat real, whole foods, and your body will thank you for it.

– FerrignKNOW TIP –
Next grocery store run, be sure to place Ferrigno FIT's top three diet-friendly items in your cart: balsamic vinegar (it adds a pop of low-calorie flavor to veggies and salads), in-shell nuts (their protein and fiber keep you satiated), and 0% plain yogurt (a creamy, comforting source of protein). Plus, Greek yogurt also works wonders as a natural low-calorie base for dressings and dips – or as a tangier alternative to sour cream.

Get to know the spice section in your local grocery store and begin using spices to replace salt. Experiment with different herbs and spices. Read the labels to ensure they are not loaded with salt. Ditch the oil and add flavor by sautéing foods in chicken broth and low-sodium soy sauce.

HERE ARE 8 WAYS TO BEAT THOSE SUGAR CRAVINGS EVERY DAY:

1. BALANCING BLOOD SUGAR

FOCUS: Do not skip meals. Keeping your blood sugar levels stabilized throughout the day is the first step to beating those cravings. If your blood sugar drops too much or sky rockets, it will make you crave a soft drink or sugary doughnut for that quick fix.

INVEST: Be careful with low-carbohydrate diets. These diets often create cravings for sweets and starches because your brain prefers running on glucose that is supplied by carbohydrates. There are good carbohydrates and bad carbohydrates – good carbs include fruits and vegetables, whole grains, whole foods.

TAKE ACTION: Eat MINI-MEALS every 3-4 hours that include protein and fiber. Choose a protein source like chicken, fish, tuna, egg whites, or nuts and add vegetables or fruit. The best part is good fats like nuts, avocados, and salmon protect your heart and support your overall health.

2. MORE WHOLE FOODS

FOCUS: Bad carbohydrates include highly processed foods that include most everything in the center aisles of the grocery store. When you do not fuel your body with enough good carbohydrates, your body craves nutrient-dense foods and if it doesn't get it, cravings for sugar can take over.

INVEST: The worst carbohydrate sources use highly refined grains and sugars. The best carbohydrates, besides fruits and vegetables, have whole or minimally processed grains. Choose whole-grain products. **One way to identify a good carbohydrate source is to divide the number of grams of carbohydrate per serving by the number of grams of fiber – aim for less than 10 for breads**

and under five for cereal.

TAKE ACTION: Spend some time in the produce section and build a mini meal around one or more whole foods like a sweet potato, whole grains, vegetables, salad, or other leafy greens. Add colorful vegetables to every meal with a touch of healthy fats from nuts, olive oil, and macadamia nut oil. Always add a good quality protein source.

3. QUALITY PROTEIN

FOCUS: Choose good quality protein. Good quality protein supports muscle and the more muscle you have, the more calories you burn just sitting here reading this book. Protein slows down the release of carbohydrates into the bloodstream and keeps blood sugar levels stable. Processed foods spike blood sugar and cause sugar cravings, so build a meal around protein and fiber.

INVEST: It is time to invest in your body by eating non-processed foods. By eating "alive" whole foods, you will be naturally detoxing your body. Foods like fresh fruits and vegetables are loaded with enzymes to help digest your food.

TAKE ACTION: Make a point of having complete meals **every 3-4 hours** throughout your day that include:

60% CARBOHYDRATES – leafy greens, salad, vegetables

20% PROTEIN – chicken, turkey, fish, tuna, 1 egg with egg whites, hummus

20% FAT – olive oil, nuts, seeds, nut butters

If you eat a meal with nothing but carbohydrates, they will be digested quickly, spiking blood sugar. Protein and good fats will sustain blood sugar and prevent cravings for sugar. Plus, it will be more difficult to get results from your workout if you are not getting enough protein at each meal.

4. TABLE SALT

FOCUS: Be aware of your salt intake. Restaurants are notorious for offering meals with high sodium content. Studies are showing that salt does damage to the arteries within 30 minutes of consumption. Limit your salt intake to no more than 2,000 mg. per day (equivalent to 1 teaspoon of salt).

INVEST: Use Himalayan Pink Salt for seasoning foods at home as it will not elevate blood pressure. Cakes, cookies, pies, chips, crackers, cheese, cured meats, dips, condiments and canned soups are full of salt, so you want to avoid them.

TAKE ACTION: Read the labels and find alternatives to limit your salt intake. Use low-sodium broths and replace the salt shaker with lemon-pepper or sea vegetable sprinkles such as dulse or nori found in the Asian food section or try gomashio (sesame salt) – a condiment made from toasted sesame seeds ground with unrefined sea salt. Himalayan Pink Salt is also a good staple to use because it does not elevate your blood pressure. It is full of minerals and is easily dissolved in the bloodstream.

5. REFINED FOODS

FOCUS: Are you eating too many refined foods? Refined foods lack nutrients and fiber, signaling the brain for more food or sugar.

INVEST: This is where the importance of time and researching ingredients comes into play. The little time you invest into what is going in your cabinets will decide what's going into your body and the energy you will have throughout the day

TAKE ACTION: Replace processed foods with more whole foods at each meal. Protein and fiber meals will fill you up and dessert may not even occur to you!

6. SUGAR INTAKE

FOCUS: Do you start your day with sugar? Take time to add up how much sugar is in every meal/snack you are eating throughout the day.

INVEST: Sugar makes you crave more sugar by stimulating your appetite: the more you eat, the more you want.

TAKE ACTION: Find healthy alternatives to satisfy your sweet tooth like yogurt, oats, and raisins mixed together for a quick, satisfying snack. Eat an apple with 1½ tablespoons of almond butter. When making puddings, pies or custards, replace sugar in the recipe with date sugar made from pure dried-powdered dates sold in health food stores.

7. STRESS EATING

FOCUS: Be honest with yourself: do you soothe emotional problems or stress with sweets?

INVEST: We are all exposed to stress each and every day and since you can't always stop stressful situations from occurring, you can support your body with good nutrition to help you handle them as they arise. Reaching for cookies, cakes, pies, caffeine, and sugar will make things worse by causing more aches and pains, indigestion, and excess body fat, which will lead to more health problems down the road.

TAKE ACTION: The key to getting lean and staying that way is to learn positive coping skills. If work is stressing you out, take a 10-minute walk instead of hitting up the cookie tray in the break room. Take a yoga class at the end of a long week. Use deep breaths to get through a phone call with your mother. And schedule time to treat yourself to a stress-less day.

8. ADRENAL GLANDS

FOCUS: Do you know where your adrenal glands are in your body?

INVEST: If the adrenal glands are exhausted, they can contribute to cravings for sugar as well as caffeine, alcohol or salt.

TAKE ACTION: Support the adrenal glands with a good-quality B-complex supplement. You can look for B-complex stress formula supplements, or you can also get plenty of B vitamins by eating leafy greens and whole grains.

WHY DINNER IS THE MOST IMPORTANT MEAL OF THE DAY

Every time you put food in your mouth, you should have three things: a table, a plate, and a chair.

Many different experts will agree that breakfast is the most important meal of the day. While I agree with this on a physical level of importance (revving up your metabolism, curbing cravings for the day, etc.) on an emotional sabotage level, dinner is just as, if not, the most important meal of the day. Both are very important for achieving your health and nutrition goals, and for keeping you on track.

Having your dinner mapped out in your head and ingredients in the fridge will help you from emotionally over eating at night. A long, hard day can result in talking yourself into that extra glass of wine or extra plate of carbs to comfort you because you "deserve it" for having a shitty boss who never hears anything you have to say.

Serve dinner from the stove by portioning out your meal first, instead of serving family-style.

If you want seconds, make sure you are conscious about it. Instead of picking from the table unconsciously, make the effort to walk to the stove.

Eating dinner early and getting to bed at a decent hour can help prevent overeating at night. Night-eating syndrome is linked with obesity, according to a review published in 2012 "Obesity Reviews." Early dinners can help you lose weight if you reduce your total calorie intake. However, going to bed hungry is unnecessary — and even counterproductive — for successful weight loss.

WEIGHT-LOSS BASICS

Regardless of the time you eat dinner, your total calorie intake determines how much weight loss you will experience.

Aim to reduce your daily intake by 500 to 1,000 calories daily to lose 1 to 2 pounds weekly, suggest the Centers for Disease Control and Prevention.

For most women, eating 1,000 to 1,600 calories a day works well for weight loss, while 1,200- to 1,600-calorie meal plans are usually effective for weight loss in men, reports the National Heart, Lung, and Blood Institute.

— FerrigKNOW TIP —
When going to the grocery store, consider paying with cash. It will help you stay on budget and limit the junk in your cart.

Timing and Size

The timing of your dinner — and other meals and snacks — is important during your weight loss venture. Consume small, frequent meals throughout the day, suggests MayoClinic.com.Eating small portions every few hours is a good rule of thumb, which can help increase your metabolism and reduce your risk for overeating.

Prepare For Snacking When You Are Not At Home — Try keeping a small bag of almonds, an apple or orange on you for when hunger strikes. If you're going to eat, at least you'll have something healthy available as opposed to running through a fast food restaurant. If you choose a protein bar, look for one containing at least 15 grams of protein and low in sugar or sweetened naturally. This may seem like a hassle at first, but you're changing your lifestyle. The more you practice this, the easier it'll be.

Eat Dinner, Or A Snack, A Few Hours Before Bedtime To Avoid Late-Night Hunger — There is nothing worse than going to bed hungry; not to mention, it makes it impossible to sleep when your stomach is growling. Eating a proper dinner at a reasonable hour that is high in protein and fiber will keep you full well into the wee hours and it will help you avoid late-night snacking.

What Is Your Relationship With Dinners? — Do you eat standing up? Watching TV? Rush through it and not make conversation while you are looking at your phone or new emails that just came in from work that you "have to take?" Take time to sit down and enjoy your meal without sitting in front of the TV.

Composition Of Meals

In addition to the size and timing of your dinner, the composition of the meal affects weight loss. Boosting your protein intake not only keeps you feeling full longer from fewer calories, but it also helps your body burn more calories. This can enhance weight loss, according to a review published in 2009 in the "Journal of Nutrition."

Eating protein at dinner will help prevent you from feeling hungry right before bed or in the middle of the night. Protein-rich foods include chicken, seafood, egg whites, cottage cheese, low-fat milk and yogurt, legumes, nuts, and seeds.

Importance Of Sleep

According to the 2012 review published in "Obesity Reviews," late-night eating is linked with insomnia and can prevent you from getting a full night's rest. Get to bed at a reasonable hour — and avoid binge eating before bed — to increase your chance of effective weight loss. Getting too-little sleep can alter appetite-regulating hormones and lead to an increased overall calorie intake, according to a review published in 2010 in "Environmental Health Perspectives." Getting seven to eight hours of sleep each night helps control appetite, and is associated with less weight gain compared with getting just five hours of sleep nightly.

Tips for Holidays, Parties, and Birthdays

Celebrations are a part of life and if you are like most people, you may put on a pound or two before New Year's Eve. Unfortunately, these extra pounds add up over the years and contribute to obesity in adults. However, it doesn't have to be that way. Portion control is the key. In other words, it is possible to enjoy your favorite foods by eating smaller portions. Here are some tips and suggestions for avoiding weight gain during the holidays and other celebrations:

Do NOT Go To A Party Hungry – If you arrive at a party starving, you may end up camping out at the buffet table. Enjoy a nutritious snack and drink some water before heading out the door.

It Is Not About The Food – Enjoy the conversation with people at the event or party instead of focusing on the food.

Chew Slowly – Learn to pace yourself when you go to a party. By chewing more slowly, you will be able to feel full with less food.

Set A Limit – Especially when it comes to hors d'ouevres. Decide how many you will have ahead of time and stick to it. Another trick I use is to hold my clutch purse in one hand and a plate or napkin of food in the other so I never have both hands free to indulge.

Use A Salad Plate Instead Of A Dinner Plate – This will help put you in control at the buffet table. Do not stack your food and watch out for dips and sauces. Fill up on fresh fruits, vegetables and shrimp cocktail.

Avoid Drinking Too Much Alcohol – You will not have as much control over what you eat if you overdo the alcohol. I like to start a party with a sparkling water and end with one before leaving an event; this not only helps hydrate you but it gives you time to say your goodbyes while setting a limit on drinks.

Be Selective At The Sweets Table – If you know you can stop at one bite, then you are better off taking a small portion of one single dessert as opposed to filling your plate up with several treats.

Be Creative With Leftovers

Leftovers are a delicious and great way to save money while you enjoy a gourmet meal the next day. You can save on calories by cutting your entrée in half and saving the other half for a meal the following day. It can be quite enjoyable to slice up some remaining steak and serve it over some mixed greens with toasted almonds or pine nuts and a bit of shaved Parmesan. Leftover vegetables can make an amazing omelet, or puree them to add into soups for a more nutrient-dense meal.

Plus, leftovers can make your life easier for the week ahead. Create a meal with leftovers and place it in an airtight container for a meal that is ready to go in the freezer. Roast vegetables and store them in an airtight container to complete a meal any night of the week. Having the right foods around in your refrigerator and freezer make it easy to eat "real" food every day.

GUIDE TO BUILDING NEW HABITS

Lasting weight loss demands you transform your eating and exercise habits. But many other choices you make each day, such as how much time you spend sleeping or surfing the Internet, can also make a difference. It is important to set small, realistic goals.

For example, getting back to the dress size you were when you were in high school might mean you need to lose over 50 pounds. A more realistic goal would be to lose 10% of your current weight with plenty of time to reach your goal. Set specific goals in the short-term, such as:

- Cooking chicken breast and roasting vegetables on your Reset day for the week ahead
- Bring your lunch to work instead of going out to lunch every day
- Go for a walk every day
- Avoid buying cookies or high-sugar foods
- Eat slowly
- Do not skip meals

Make these habits a routine. Once you are consistent with one or more of these habits, add one more. Over time, you will see how they are all connected and will lead to successful weight loss. Make a plan to stick with it for at least a week and you will also realize it is much easier to do than you might think.

Eating Like Europeans

Allow culture to be your guide, not science.

Eating healthy and well, not dieting, is the key to achieving and maintaining successful weight loss. "Dieting" (notice the first three letters spell "die") or feeling deprived will not get you where you want to go. How food makes you feel (energized) and how it tastes is the secret to eating well. Europeans take pleasure in eating well while Americans tend obsess over it and see it as a conflict.

Europeans think about eating "good food" while Americans, especially women, worry about 'bad food' to eat. Though the French have lots of saturated fat and alcohol in their diets, they are not an obese country because they eat small portions, no seconds or snacking and they take pleasure when they eat communal meals.

When Americans hear the terms "eating well," many still associate these words with "dieting," weight loss and most foods being off-limits or do not taste good. It can make us feel worse about ourselves if we view our weight problems because we can't stick with a "diet." How do we get away from this negative type of thinking, enjoy our food and feel good about ourselves?

Ask Yourself: Do Any Of These Situations Apply To Me?

- I eat out all the time
- I only bring prepared food home to eat
- I eat really fast
- I generally watch TV or read when eating
- I belong to the "clean the plate" club regardless if I am hungry or not
- I rarely walk anywhere — and love my car

If any or all of these sound familiar, you are a typical American eater. Europeans walk every day to the market to purchase fresh ingredients to cook a meal. They use spices and fresh herbs to create flavorful meals and serve small portions that are quite tasty. A glass of wine is enjoyed over a leisurely meal and is often finished with a piece of dark chocolate or fresh fruit.

RETHINK HEALTHY EATING

Instead of focusing on weight loss and dieting, think about being healthy. Take note of when you feel hungry and when you feel full as you eat. Be aware of portion sizes and stop eating when you are full. Do some sort of physical activity every day — think of it as doing something just for you. Feed yourself on a regular schedule and try new foods, choosing quality over quantity. Think about what you are eating and savor every bite. Reset that palate!

CLIENT STORY: KATY

A woman named Katy came to see me a few years ago. She was 48 and a mother of two. Her eldest daughter had just moved away to college and her son, being 16, had just gotten his driver's license. She had been married to her husband Ralph, a financial advisor, since they had graduated college at ASU. Katy came to me because she said after her son Michael was born she was never able to take off all the weight she intended to. With her eldest Bella, she was able to get back into shape after only a couple of months. Katy was 5'6" and, as a kid, never had any issues with weight. She was involved in sports, the debate club, and was a photographer for the school's newspaper. She stayed involved in these activities until she graduated college. She worked as a paralegal until a month before giving birth to Bella.

Six months after Bella was born, Ralph's father was killed in a car accident, leaving Ralph's mother on her own. Ralph's career was taking off and instead of going back to work, Katy decided to remain a stay-at-home mom to be there for her mother-in-law. A year later, Katy got pregnant with Michael. She spoke to me about loving her children and was proud to be a stay-at-home mom.

Katy had friends, but her life was dedicated to her kids through the PTA, being classroom mom and all-around chauffer for every activity they became interested in. Though Ralph provided a good life financially for them, he lived at the office. Over the years, Katy became lonely, and it was only when she looked back she could finally admit it. Katy loved sweets and made it a nightly habit to eat her cookies in bed. If the kids got ice cream, pizza or cake, so would she. Food was one of her favorite ways to bond with her kids.

Two months before she came to see me, she said she had walked into her house and the silence was deafening to her. Not only was no one home, but there was no one to pick up from school, no fighting, no laughter and no one to cook dinner for. She knew she had been in denial for a while, but it didn't sink in until that moment. She had gained over 40 pounds since marrying her husband and admitted to giving up on her appearance completely. Though Ralph was addicted to work he was still in love with Katy. Katy loved Ralph but she wanted to learn to love herself again. When he came home late that night, they talked for hours. Katy was coming to terms with the fact that though she loved her life raising her children, as a stay-at-home mom, they were not going to need her the same way as when they were young. Katy was lost and she had to figure out what her third act in life was going to look like.

I explained to her about the third act scenario. Most plays have two acts and, a hundred years ago, many people did not live past 60 years old. I have clients who train with me and are in great health well into their 80s. This third act is the "choice act." It was time for Katy to figure out what she wanted to do in her last act of life and examine what she could do now that her kids were independent. Katy decided she would get back into shape so that anything she wanted to do she wouldn't hesitate to do.

Katy and I began working together. I put her on *The Reset Plan* and she kept conquering every one of her habits over those 66 days. She kept repeating new habits until, eventually, they became a lifestyle. Over time, instead of thinking how sad and lonely it was cooking for two, she began examining new, decadent recipes. She took the time to enjoy them with all five of her senses. She spent endless hours a week at the local grocers, buying produce for her latest recipes. She brought back her photography skills and started a food blog with a friend she met at a spinning class. When we worked together we never concentrated on losing weight but instead on gaining back a lifestyle that suited her now.

I saw Katy a few months back at a local farmers market. She looked fantastic. She was lean and her energy was infectious. We talked about how much we both dislike the taste of blueberries, but how healthy they are because of their antioxidants. The greatest piece of news was that her entire family was getting ready to hike Machu Picchu together to celebrate Michael graduating high school.

What I love most about Katy was that she didn't try to change her husband and his lifestyle at work, nor guilt her kids into paying more attention to her. Instead of being depressed, she made a plan to take action. I admire Katy and was proud I helped her become her own personal trainer. I know she will get to the top of that mountain first.

EXCUSE #3:
I DON'T HAVE ENOUGH TIME TO WORK OUT

This is probably the most popular excuse I hear from my clients: "I don't have enough time to work out."

This excuse makes me cringe every time I hear it... which is constantly. Sometimes a few more hours in a day would be nice but it's never going to happen, so the trick is to start getting organized and prioritize your daily activities. Be honest with yourself: is it you don't have enough time, or is it you don't want to make time? It's human nature for most people to do only what they absolutely need to do to get by. Some might call this lazy, but I understand it's efficient and instinctual. If this is your natural instinct, you must fight against it in the case of working out.

Even if your doctor prescribes an exercise program or if you are taking medication, exercise is a must. If you have exercised before, you may have noticed your energy levels increased, you could think more clearly and sleep better. Many of my clients tell me they feel less anxious, enjoy a sense of well-being, get strong, and, of course, lose weight. Regular exercise is one of the best ways to prevent depression and reduce the risk of health issues and disease.

Part of your game-change here will be mental because you need to learn to prioritize your body's need for exercise in the same way you would prioritize the health and well-being of your family members or the needs of your boss and colleagues. Forget the idea that you are "wasting" time working out. Ask yourself how much time and how many opportunities you have wasted if you are unfit and/or overweight.

Ask yourself how much time will be wasted on medical appointments and treatment if and when you experience a health crisis. Your fitness is important. If you are a generally well-functioning person, I bet you usually show up for the appointments you make with other people. You need to give yourself that same respect and keep the exercise appointments you make with yourself.

When I train clients I applaud them as they walk into my door. Showing up for life and keeping your commitments is a winning mentality, and with working out, showing up is more than half the battle. If a client shows up on a day where they are feeling "off," even better — it's important to acknowledge that. But you can usually work around it while still listening to your body.

Remember: before you begin exercising, make sure you have arranged for a physical examination, especially if you have any health issues, have been sedentary for quite some time or are over the age of 60. If you have been exercising and realize it is not enough, gradually increase the intensity. The body is able to adapt better when gradual change in exercise is incorporated. Plus, you will not be as sore, especially if you overdo it the first few times you meet with a trainer or try a new routine.

You can also add exercise to your daily routine. Park further away from your workplace, for example, and walk those extra steps or take the stairs instead of the elevator. If you already go for a walk every day, add ten more minutes to your walk. Determine what exercise is going to fit into your schedule. How are you going to make exercise a part of your daily life?

THE RIGHT EXERCISE PROGRAM FOR YOU

Find an exercise you enjoy and can look forward to. If you like to exercise alone, I would try yoga, swimming, or hiking. A daily bike ride might be just the ticket. If you prefer team sports, you may want to join your local softball or bowling league. Any kind of exercise is acceptable; however, for best results, incorporating weight training is the most efficient way to lose body fat, keep muscle, and enhance your performance in other exercises.

Make a list of exercises you are going to do. If you are going to weight train, make a list of other options and post it in a place that is convenient for you. Every day, decide how you are going to exercise. If the weather is bad and you usually go for a walk, then put some music on and dance to your favorite tunes.

Simply Walk

Walking needs to get some extra attention here because it really is the most convenient form of exercise for most people. It works well because all you need are a pair of good walking shoes. It doesn't cost anything and there are plenty of places to walk, such as your local park, sidewalks, or the track at your local high school. Take the time to enjoy being outside and connect with nature. You don't really need special clothes either, as you can walk in pretty much whatever you are wearing that day.

Shoe-shop in the evening; your feet swell during the day and stop in the late afternoon, so you want to shop when they're at their biggest. Also make sure the sneakers are a little roomy — enough so that you can wiggle your toes, but no more than that. They should be comfy from the get-go.

Sticking To It

Many people struggle with sticking with an exercise program. You might feel that your schedule is too hectic or it interferes with your family life. Here are some strategies that will help you get over this hurdle:

- Think of exercise as "play" time
- Find an exercise buddy or exercise with a family member or friend
- Put aside a dollar for every day that you exercise and save it for a new outfit or massage — after a while you will find out that exercise itself is reward enough.
- Focus on positive thoughts when you exercise
- Schedule it — this provides structure and ensures your exercise program continues
- Invest in an exercise bike or Pilates machine so you can watch television while you exercise

If you miss a day, do *not* give up or stop exercising. If you get a flat tire on your car, you don't flatten the other tires. You fix the tire and keep going. If you happen to have an illness or injury and have to stop exercising, begin again gradually. The benefits of exercise are endless. If you still think to yourself that nothing works, make note of how you feel after you exercise. This can be a strong motivator to keep going no matter what.

If you think you're too busy to exercise, try this experiment: For one day, schedule a time to work out, and then stick to it — even if you can exercise for only 10 minutes. At the end of the day, ask yourself if you were any less productive than usual. The answer will probably be no — and your favorite excuse will be gone.

Success happens when your dreams get bigger than your excuses.

The Importance of Consistency

Let's face it: most of our daily lives are rather habitual, meaning you do the same thing day in and day out. Our daily habits, whether they are good or bad, make us who we are. The key to success is controlling them when it comes to weight loss. Knowing how to form positive habits and ditching the negative ones will help you see changes in your physique. A small effort makes a huge difference. If you don't like an exercise, start doing it. You're probably avoiding it because you're weak and out of practice.

I have been doing this for years by revamping my diet, exercising daily, and making every effort to move more and sit less. The littlest changes can improve the quality of life, more than you realize.

Focus On One Change For The Next 30 Days

After the first 30 days, enough time will have passed to sufficiently condition your body for a positive, new healthy habit. One of the best ways to start a new habit is to replace lost needs. For example, if you need to be consistent with exercise, try signing up for a class that meets on a regular basis.

However, if the change you make causes more pain than joy, it will be difficult to stick with it. If you are someone who hates going to the gym for your workout, then find an exercise you enjoy doing and look forward to — you might feel more comfortable in a Pilates studio or you just might want to train on your own.

Write your goals down and clarify what the changes you are going to make will mean to you. Embrace the idea of doing a little bit and build on that success. It will help you stay committed to your fitness goals, making them more difficult to dismiss. Be patient and know most new habits go through a series of barriers or changes in your life. Give yourself a reward if you have successfully changed a habit or ditched a negative one to give you an extra push. Keep it simple and make sure your habit is as consistent as possible.

There is no better way to break negative habits than having the confidence to do so. Confidence is key to living a healthy life.

Get Rid Of The Scale

The scale tells you nothing about your health. The number on the scale says nothing about whether you're moving in the right direction with your health and leaves you with PTDD (Post Traumatic Diet Disorder). Many things may affect the number on the scale: the time of day that you weigh yourself, hormone levels, or even what you recently ate or drank. Women especially seem to think it is the ultimate indicator of failure or success and that is simply not true. Muscle weighs more than fat — well, actually, one pound of fat weighs the same as a pound of muscle, but the muscle is more condensed than the fat. In other words, if you lost ten pounds of fat and replaced it with ten pounds of muscle, you might weigh the same, but you will look and feel better. The scale is not the best motivator to continue eating healthy and exercising. In fact, if the number you want to see does not appear on the scale, you can feel very discouraged and disappointed.

When you get rid of the scale, you can measure your progress by how you feel and look, and how your clothes are fitting. This is definitely more fun. The wrong number on the scale can set you up to feel terrible; do not give the scale any power over you. In fact, getting rid of the scale can help you avoid the all-or-nothing mentality and the obsession with the numbers game. Eating healthy and exercising is what will help you feel great and generally take care of yourself. Perfection is not sustainable over the long haul, but looking and feeling good is. By focusing on this, you will naturally lose weight. You want your healthy weight to be a place you can maintain long-term. It is not fair to compare your current weight to your past weight; again, focus on how much healthier you feel, and work hard to improve that instead of focusing on the scale. Instead of the scale, ask yourself:

- How do I feel?
- Do I feel healthy?
- Do I have more energy?
- Am I regularly moving my body and doing exercise I enjoy?
- Are my strength and endurance improving?
- Am I generally choosing foods that nourish my body and make me feel good?
- Am I listening to my body's hunger cues?
- How do my clothes fit? Am I remembering to love my body exactly as it is?

The Benefits of Having Muscle

One of the best benefits for having more muscle is that it allows you to help ease the pain of arthritis, obesity, diabetes, and back pain. Weight-bearing exercises also help build bone density to prevent osteoporosis. Increased muscle mass means more strength, making it easier to perform routine daily tasks.

Muscle makes you look lean and toned, allowing your clothes to fit better even if you do not lose weight. Plus, the more muscle you have, the more calories you burn. Adding more muscle to your body can make you burn more calories at rest. Fat burns very few calories because it does not do anything to help your body move. You can actually burn 15% more calories per day by adding more muscle.

– FerrigKNOW TIP –

Dread long workouts? Then don't do them! Keep your weight workouts under an hour. After 60 minutes, your body starts producing more of the stress hormone cortisol, which can have a testosterone-blocking, muscle-wasting effect.

If You Are Eating Out, Ask For a Box In Advance

When you are eating out it's important to make a game plan in advance and stick with it. Focus on making healthy choices at restaurants, no matter what. Get in the habit of ordering water because calories from other drinks can add up quickly. Do not start mindlessly eating the bread basket; save your calories for your meal. Choose lean meats like chicken or fish and have it grilled, steamed, baked or broiled instead of fried. Salads and vegetables should be a part of your meal.

To avoid overeating or belonging to the clean-the-plate club, order a few small plates from the appetizer menu. If you do order an entrée, ask for a to-go container when it is served and cut your food in half to save for another meal. A great trick that helps me is looking at the menu in advance. It relieves the anxiety of figuring out what to order while trying to have a conversation and allows me to order first which sets the bar for the table and doesn't allow me to be tempted by anyone else's order.

If you find meal prepping hard this week, or cooking almost impossible with your tight schedule, be prepared to "improvise" and assemble your meals. At this point you have no excuses not to have fresh food in your fridge. Tuna, balsamic vinegar and walnuts make a great go-to meal in a pinch.

Remember, you cannot out-work a bad diet.

TIPS FOR GETTING THE MOST OUT OF YOUR WORKOUTS

You can totally waste your time if you do not make a plan when going to the gym. Set clear training goals when you go to the gym so you don't wander around aimlessly from one piece of equipment to another. Figure out the best time for you to go to the gym and exercise. There is no "right" time to exercise, but consistency is key.

Try to find a workout partner: according to Michigan State University research, exercising with someone who's in better shape than you can help you work out 208% longer. Don't be intimidated or jealous of someone in better shape; join forces and encourage each other. Your bodies will thank you.

Performing the same exercises day after day will lead you to a plateau rather quickly, bringing any progress to a complete halt. One of the best ways to avoid plateauing is to keep a workout log where you can record the exercises, weight, repetitions, and sets during each training session. Use this information to create and add new exercises that will challenge you.

BUILD At A Fast Rate: Work opposing muscle groups — your biceps and triceps, for instance — back-to-back for a faster workout. While one muscle is working, the other is forced to rest. You won't need as much time between sets.

However, you do not want to risk injury. Try to meet with a professional for a training session that will allow you to learn the "do's and dont's" from the start. Learning new exercises can boost your performance and motivation. Between sets, take 20 to 30 seconds to stretch the muscle you just worked. Boston researchers found that women and men who followed this stretching pattern increased their strength by 20 percent. Of course, warming up is an important part of every workout. Stick to warm-ups that match the workout you've planned, priming your body for the work ahead.

Using proper form is critical in preventing injury and getting results. For example, if you are doing squats, make sure you stand tall with your chest lifted, shoulders back and down and your core muscles engaged. Keep a soft bend in the knee while you shift your weight into your heels. Use a bench to squat with perfect form. That is, stand in front of the bench when you squat. Lower yourself as if you were sitting down. When your butt touches the bench, push yourself back up. Try it with a light bar or a broomstick first.

We have great tips at FerrignoFIT.com. For example, you can recover faster from a hard workout by lightly exercising the same muscles the following day. Use light weight — about 20 percent of the weight you can lift one time — and do two sets of 25 repetitions. This will deliver more blood and nutrients into your muscles so they repair faster.

If they are supportive, let your family and friends know about your workout goals. They can contribute a lot toward keeping you motivated. One way to enhance your workouts is to consider signing up for a contest or race of some sort. Another option might be to compete against the clock by performing as many push-ups or sit-ups in one minute. It never hurts to have a bigger goal in mind. However, when it comes to exercise, aim for being fit, not perfect. Put your trust in regular workouts, not the latest product for weight loss.

– FerrignKNOW TIP –
Count your repetitions backward. When you near the end of the set, you'll think about how many you have left instead of how many you've done.

– FerrignKNOW TIP –
Look at your dominant hand—without turning your head—while you're bench-pressing. You'll be able to lift more weight

DEMYSTIFYING THE SPLURGE MEAL

A "splurge meal" is important to enjoy and is when you eat something not part of your regular healthy eating plan. Typically, this meal will have junk food such as hamburgers, french fries, or pizza. As long as you are following your healthy eating plan daily, you can include one or two splurge meals per week. Splurge meals are meant to satisfy your cravings or taste buds, not binge on an all-you-can-eat buffet. It does not mean you can splurge all day long — only a single meal. By limiting yourself to a single meal, splurging will not derail your results or prevent you from losing weight.

Eating a splurge meal can help boost your metabolism but it can also help you psychologically. It is difficult to eat "clean" all the time, seven days a week. A splurge meal allows you to stay sane and stay in the game. Plan your splurge meal and most likely you will notice you do not feel as energized as you're now used to — or, in some cases, even nauseous. When you eat clean all week and then eat a splurge meal, your body may respond negatively, such as, "What is going on?" When you eat healthy, whole foods, the body knows exactly what to do with all those powerful nutrients — another motivator for eating healthy.

SIGN UP FOR A FITNESS EVENT

You will be amazed how committed you will feel when you have an event coming up to get ready for. In fact, any time you change up your normal workout, it can help maximize results. For example, if you normally walk, try jogging every few minutes for a minute or two. If you are already are a runner, add some short sprints into your run. Try something completely new, like cycling or Zumba class. Shocking your body with something new can lead to amazing results.

ADD TWO NEW MOVES TO YOUR WORKOUT PLAN

Any type of strength training is going to help you increase muscle mass. For example, yoga and Pilates help strengthen your core muscles, including your back, by lengthening and strengthening. It is *not* a good idea to carry hand weights or wear ankle weights while you are walking or running, as they can damage your joints. Of course, it is important to get plenty of cardiovascular exercise to get your heart rate up. Cardiovascular exercise can include walking, hiking, running, or taking an aerobics or dance class; you can also use the cardio equipment at your local gym, or try kickboxing.

Aim for 30-40 minutes of cardiovascular exercise at least 4-5 times per week. You should be able to carry on a conversation while doing your cardio work. Be consistent with the schedule, add variety to your workouts including intensity, and you will definitely see results. Try to train with a dumbbell weight that equals the amount of weight you have already lost. It's not only a great reminder and motivation, but it's truly empowering to make gains with the weight in the right way.

THE IMPORTANCE OF MUSCLE – PHYSICALLY

Stroke and heart disease are still the leading causes of death in the United States. However, you can reduce the risk of heart disease and other health conditions by increasing physical activity. Regular exercise helps you lower blood pressure and cholesterol levels and reduces the risk of developing Type 2 diabetes and metabolic syndrome. Metabolic syndrome is a condition with a combination of factors including:

- Too much body fat around the waist
- Low HDL (good) cholesterol
- High triglycerides
- High blood sugar

The more physical activity you do, the lower your risk of metabolic syndrome will be.

If you already have Type 2 diabetes, regular exercise can help control blood glucose levels every single day. Regular exercise also helps lower your risk of many types of cancer, including breast and colon cancer. It is possible to improve your quality of life as well as physical fitness.

As we get older, it is important to strengthen our muscles, joints, and bones. They support the body and make it easier to move. Doing strength-training and aerobic exercise go a long way in strengthening bones, muscles and joints, and preventing osteoporosis. Muscle-strengthening exercises can help you maintain strength and muscle mass. Increasing the amount of weight you lift and the number of repetitions in a slow, consistent manner will give you endless health benefits, not matter how old you are.

Improves Your Mood and Mental Health

Regular exercise improves your judgment, thinking, and learning skills. Plus, it can help you sleep better and reduce your risk of depression. Performing a mix of cardiovascular exercise and muscle-strength training at least 3-5 times per week offers many mental health benefits. Being strong, healthy, and lean will go a long way in improving your mood and mental health.

Prevents Falling

Being physically active makes it easier to do daily activities like grocery shopping, climbing stairs, and playing with pets and children. Continuing to be physically active through strength training and supporting lean muscle tissue can lower your risk of any physical limitations as you age. The fear of falling is something many older adults face, and continuing a strength training program is one of the best ways to prevent or eliminate the risk of falling.

The # 1 Anti-Aging Secret

Do you want to increase your chances of living longer? Exercise is the number one way to slow down the aging process from the inside out. Regular physical activity has a huge impact on your health. Studies show people who are physically active at least seven hours per week have a 40% less chance of dying early than those who are physically active for less than thirty minutes per week.

Everyone benefits from regular physical activity – size, shape, ethnicity and age do not matter.

THE IMPORTANCE OF MUSCLE – MENTALLY

Staying strong with plenty of muscle not only keeps you strong and healthy physically, but it also boosts brain function. Regardless of your age, studies continue to show regular exercise and staying strong lead to healthier lives overall. Here are the mental benefits of keeping muscle and being physically fit:

Reduces Stress – Increases norepinephrine, a chemical in the brain that can help slow down the stress response.

Creates Feelings Of Happiness — Exercise gives you endorphins. Endorphins create feelings of happiness and are a great way to prevent depression.

Boosts Self-Esteem — Regardless of your weight, size, or shape, exercise can improve your perception of attractiveness and positive self-image.

Prevents Degenerative Diseases Of The Brain — Regular exercise helps to prevent cognitive decline. Exercise boosts the chemicals in the brain that support and prevent degeneration of the hippocampus — an important part of the brain for learning and memory.

Relieves Anxiety — The chemicals released in the brain after exercise can actually calm you down and reduce or alleviate anxiety.

Creates New Brain Cells — Studies continue to show regular cardiovascular exercise can create new brain cells and improve overall brain function.

Supports Addiction Recovery — Dopamine is a chemical in the brain released in response to any form of pleasure such as food, sex, drugs or alcohol.

Exercise can actually help addicts of drugs or alcohol, for example, to de-prioritize cravings.

Reboots The Body Clock — A moderate workout can serve as a natural sleeping aid, especially for those with insomnia. Exercise raises your body temperature, so when your body temperature goes back to normal afterwards, this signals the body that it is time to sleep.

Be More Productive — Regular exercise allows you to be more productive, creative, and have more energy. Going for a walk or weight-training session helps clear the mind and body at the same time.

— FerrigKNOW TIP —
Research shows that listening to music when you exercise can produce positive thoughts and help offset fatigue. Put together a playlist that makes you feel like moving.

Sometimes it takes a while to uncover your secret. In the meantime, you can commit to stop making excuses, start showing up, and prioritize your fitness. Finding time to work out is never about finding additional time for your training. It is about finding how that time can fit into your existing schedule.

This is going to sound old-school, but get a whiteboard or an old-fashioned calendar book and go over your weekly schedule with an eye towards fitting in some exercise. Don't only put the exercise appointments into your phone, even if you need to do this as well. Write them out to commit to them. Cross them off when they are executed. Most people find something rewarding about using a hard calendar for tracking daily exercise goals and food. I encourage you to give this a try and see if it works for you.

Think hard about when you schedule your workouts. By the end of the day, many of us use the excuse: "I'm too tired to exercise." I understand this and am a fan of exercising before work when it is possible. This can actually benefit you in multiple ways. Getting your workout in early in the day will not only release endorphins, wake you up, and promote better circulation, it will help you knock out your daily exercise obligation and give you some additional motivation to make better food choices during the demanding workday ahead.

When you are making your exercise plans, rethink the idea of only working out by appointment in the gym or that your workouts have to last for an hour. See if there are certain things you can substitute, like a long walk or streaming fitness workouts on the days when you are going to be really slammed. Can you not leave your job long enough to take a class today? Close your office door and jump rope for 10 minutes or plan to walk on your lunch break. Start with scheduling 10 minutes, doing something active you like or focusing on a body part you want to see a change in right away. There is no such thing as spot-reducing, but 10 minutes of targeted exercise can help tighten a specific zone and make that change come faster. Think, "10 you're in!" Taking the stairs instead of the elevator or walking instead of driving are other ways to get your heart pumping — and these little things do add up.

FOCUS: Commit to solving your exercise problem this week. What are your obstacles? Change your perspective; just because you can't make it to the gym or put in an entire hour at one time doesn't mean you have to forfeit the workout completely.

INVEST: Plan ahead. Keep in mind that exercise doesn't always have to be a formal workout.

TAKE ACTION: Here are some tips and tricks I've seen be successful for my clients. See if one or more of them can help you:

- Treat yourself like you would your most important client and do not cancel your workout plans. If that's hard, find a workout buddy whom you know will keep you accountable if you cancel on them.
- Go to sleep in your workout clothes if you have to, and pack your gym bag the night before. Place your shoes by the front door.
- Place your alarm clock or phone across the room and set it to an upbeat song that motivates you and makes you want to get out of bed.
- Remind yourself that 30 minutes is 2% of your day. If you would rather spend 2% watching a TV show, fine – but don't fast forward through the commercials. Grab your weights or resistance bands and do some reps during the breaks.
- Start a score jar. Every time you don't work out put $5 in the jar. Hopefully you won't miss too many workouts, but if it is that type of week, month use the money to buy new gym gear. New clothes can motivate us to want to show them off and it makes us feel good to look good.

- For the next week wear a rubber band around your wrist. Every time you sense yourself making an excuse or being negative about working out, snap the band to remind yourself to snap out of it.
- In the same way you can "earn" your food by working out, you can connect other things you enjoy with ways of getting extra exercise. Every time you buy something on the Internet, consider doing 20 sit-ups, 20 push-ups, and 20 jumping jacks first. You may find that when you "earn" physically what you are spending financially, you spend less money. Either way, there's an upside.

You have already seen a discussion of the "diets don't work" or "I've tried everything" excuses, which leads into the focus of the first seven days, where I asked you to begin closely observing your own environment, habits, and emotions related to food and fitness. Record those observations in a journal, and begin to incorporate (or increase the amount of) walking in your day. You will use the results of your self-audit to choose a food plan from the book to start during the next seven-day period and to create an appropriate exercise plan.

During the following weeks, you will be guided to make choices within your exercise plans that will make them even more challenging and healthful, so that by the end of the last seven day period you are:

- Effectively running and/or walking on a regular basis
- Routinely doing weight training exercises and eating a balanced, moderately calorie-restricted diet of lean protein, produce, and whole-grain carbohydrates
- Significantly reducing — if not altogether eliminating — sugar, white flour, salt, preservatives, and additives

Ultimately, you are learning to become your own personal trainer.

These changes will be less painful and more sustainable than if they are undertaken in one week. You may find yourself becoming a new person following the seven day cycles. The goal is to retain a lot of self -awareness and power during *The Reset Plan* process: you are choosing your own foods, modifying your exercises, thinking and writing about your experiences, and taking control of other aspects of your life (this is the point of the small household projects). For example: have you been consistent with making your bed? Have you gotten rid of clothing in your closet you haven't worn in years?

Don't feel rushed through this process: you are free to repeat a particular seven-day week before moving on to the next. Go at your own pace. People who commit to this keep moving forward: they have experienced success (weight loss, improved fitness) and have incorporated the new behaviors gradually, on their own terms, with a great deal of attention to their patterns. The journaling helped those who have completed the plan to notice how the changes made them feel every step of the way. Another advantage of a gradual rollout is that it keeps people from getting bored. Having micro-goals each week (to increase fiber intake, reduce sugar intake, incorporate free weights, etc.) helps to divert attention from the overall reality of following a disciplined new regimen.

While each person's goals and starting points are different, by the end of twelve weeks, you will lose some weight, improve your level of fitness, develop insight about your personal challenges and strengths related to your health, and feel powerful. I know it's not as flashy as a quick weight-loss promise, but it's for real and it's sustainable. The weight losses (and fitness gains) can be much larger and longer lasting, depending on where you are and if you are ready to do the work. *The Reset Plan* will guide you every step of the way.

HERE ARE JUST A FEW OF *THE RESET PLAN* STRATEGIES YOU CAN START RIGHT AWAY:

Make time in your daily schedule for YOU — Allow for at least 10-15 minutes to go for a walk, play with your pets, enjoy your morning coffee, or take a long bath.

Review Your Day's Meals — Are they giving you the energy you need? Are you feeling lethargic or energized after a meal? Are you craving junk food or sugar? Asking these questions will help you identify the changes you need to make for the days ahead.

Write Your Goals Down — Is there a wedding or other special event in your future, or are you on the border of becoming diabetic? Post these in your bedroom, bathroom, and on the refrigerator so you will see them every day.

Embrace The Challenge Of Getting FIT — Be proud of your decision and let others know you are making changes to your lifestyle.

Think Protein And Fiber For Meals — Consuming fewer calories, especially at dinner, can help you feel full and not store those extra calories as fat. Pairing lean protein with high-fiber vegetables at each meal will do the trick.

Before You Go Out To A Restaurant — Look at their menu online and know what you are going to order before you go. The other option is to know what you are going to eat and not open the menu at all. It can be too tempting, especially if there are pictures throughout the menu.

Create A Food Preparation Day — It might be on the weekend or your day off when you can prepare grilled chicken breasts, roast some vegetables or stock up on whole foods that will fit with your meal plan.

Make A Grocery Shopping List — Keep a pad handy on your counter so you can write down the foods you need or are about to run out of. This will help you stay focused and lower your grocery bill.

Stock Your Pantry And Refrigerator With Healthy Foods — Make sure you can always grab a quick meal no matter what time of day it is. Eating healthy should not make you anxious or stressed out. Keep hard-boiled eggs handy; Greek yogurt and berries and grilled chicken breast and roasted sweet potatoes are always good options, too.

Keep Healthy Snacks Handy — When it is late afternoon and you are feeling tired and stressed, give your body some good nutrition to improve your mood. A good choice is a small apple with one tablespoon of ground almond butter.

Think "Whole Foods" — Highly processed foods are full of sugar, trans fats, sodium, preservatives, additives, and fillers. These are all bad for your health and can trigger cravings. Eating whole foods, without any of these, is the best way to prevent food addictions.

Test A Meal — Choose a meal where you need to make some improvements. For example, if you are used to skipping breakfast, try eating a healthy breakfast of protein and fiber and see if you notice a difference in how you feel. If you skip the bread at dinner and focus on eating more vegetables, do you notice you feel alert after the meal as opposed to wanting to crash on the couch?

Keep Emergency Foods On Hand — If you have a long day ahead, make sure you do not go anywhere without food. Keep a cooler in your car for fresh vegetables and hummus or stash a small bag of almonds in your computer bag.

Find Other Activities To Do Besides Eating Out — Most social gatherings revolve around food; however, you can also spend time with friends doing things that are more active.

Exercise Every Chance You Get — Take the stairs at work or wherever you can. Hold the plank position for one minute followed by ten push-ups. Make a collection of your favorite songs you can dance to. Find ways to move throughout your day.

Time Your Meals — The best way to burn body fat is to eat smaller meals no longer than 3-4 hours apart to keep your metabolism running at optimum levels. Make sure you consume adequate amounts of protein with plenty of water to support lean muscle.

The more muscle you have, the more calories you will burn reading this book.

CLIENT STORY: CLARE

A few years ago, I had a client named Clare who was about 60 pounds overweight. She came to me because she was unhappy about being unable to play with her kids at the park without constantly losing her breath. She was experiencing some back and knee pain, and was noticing how simple things like pushing her kids on the swing were a struggle.

Clare seemed somewhat downbeat but also had a hopeful spirit about her, and was open to exploring any workout method or tool I suggested — except for the scale and the treadmill. She was a soft-spoken woman until we discussed the scale and treadmill. She was adamant walking on the treadmill would hurt her knees and made it clear if I ever put her on the scale or a treadmill she would never come back to my gym again.

I treat each client as an individual and really get interested in what activity each one likes and what they can't stand to do for exercise, so I love it when clients are direct with me. What interested me the most was Clare's energy and the hardening of her eyes when she discussed the treadmill and scale; I suspected it had less to do with the actual machines, and more to do with a trauma associated with them.

Some trainers will argue with their clients and encourage them to face their fears right away, just as some parents throw their kids into the deep end of the pool to teach them how to swim. I believe being a good parent, friend, trainer, or leader requires paying attention when a person tells you who they are and respecting their fears.

For several months, Clare and I trained on programs that kept her not only off, but nowhere near, a treadmill or a scale. We walked, biked, and did the elliptical. She worked her ass off and we measured her progress by taking body measurements each week. Clare strengthened her back and saw improvement in her knees and her general muscle tone. I noticed her energy and attitude also seemed to be transforming as well.

About six months into our training, Clare came in on a Monday and enthusiastically opened up about her weekend. Clare and her family had hiked three miles. She had also played baseball with her kids without feeling tired or winded at all. She felt empowered and decided nothing was going to stand in her way again. She suggested we start our session on the treadmill. And we began to talk.

It turns out Clare had struggled with her weight as a kid. Her mother, a former beauty pageant winner, insisted Clare compete as well and envisioned it as a bonding experience for them. Clare's mother closely monitored her food intake leading up to the pageant and — you guessed it — purchased a treadmill for Clare to use in the garage. Clare and her mother would do a daily weigh-in before school and use the number on the scale to determine how long she would walk on the treadmill that day. This routine went on for weeks leading up to the competition.

According to Clare, her mother and the coach she hired would pinch her fat as "encouragement" to get the weight off. She did lose weight, but she starved herself, was bitter about the seemingly endless hours on the treadmill, and became obsessed with the scale number. Clare remembers feeling exhausted, defeated, and bitter when she was onstage and she didn't win the pageant or feel emotionally closer to her mother. When it was over, Clare began to gain weight as fast as she could, so that even if her mother tried to enter her again, it would take too long for the weight to come off for her to even stand a chance.

Clare had spent the weekend bonding with her own children through physical activity and made the connection that she never wanted to do anything that sabotaged her from being the mother she wanted to be. She needed to accept that even though she didn't have the relationship with her mother that she had wanted and needed, it didn't mean she had to run away from things — like the treadmill — that reminded her of tough times or people. This was Clare's "game on" moment. She realized, through weight training and other activities, that she really did enjoy being active and fit, for herself and for her family. She ran her first marathon a year later.

EXCUSE #4:
I CAN'T AFFORD A GYM MEMBERSHIP

While this chapter confronts two very common excuses people make to keep from exercising, it really serves to address the importance of building a community that will be supportive of your fitness goals and commitment to a healthy lifestyle. It also offers practical guidance if you want to work out at home.

You will also be guided through specific cardio and strength training "upgrades" this week, as well as challenged to begin making even healthier choices regarding protein within the parameters of your food plan. The fourth week of *The Reset Plan* offers specific guidance and detailed options for increasing cardio workouts and strength training exercises.

THE BENEFITS OF EXERCISE WITH A PARTNER, GROUP, OR ONLINE COMMUNITY

Working out with a partner, group, or online community can help you stay committed to your fitness goals and have fun at the same time. In addition to making exercise fun, working out with a partner or group helps you schedule your workouts and pull you out of a rut or work through a plateau. Having a support system that comes with a gym membership is an important factor in creating a long-term fitness success.

A gym membership provides a powerful combination of accountability, support, motivation and, in some cases, healthy competition. For example, taking classes at your local gym can play the role of a coach, cheerleader, or teammate and be worth every penny. All of the above can motivate you to do one more repetition, lift more weight, and help you keep going when you feel like quitting. It feels so much better when we are getting positive reinforcement from others, especially when it comes to work and exercise.

It is important to choose a partner who has a similar commitment to you when it comes to fitness and nutrition. You don't want to be injured, held back or pushed too hard. The person you train with does not have to be your best friend, but it is important you like each other and feel committed to that person to stay with your workouts. You can feel this way towards a fitness class, personal trainer or your workout buddy. Which arrangement works best for you? I always like working out with a partner who does one or a few things better than me. I may be great with my arm exercises but if I need that extra motivation for legs, I know my partner enjoys working them and will help get me through a killer, challenging workout.

One-On-One

Working out with a friend or colleague may work well for those who are more introverted and shy away from fitness classes or gyms. One-on-one works well if you have a specific goal such as training for an event, losing weight, or getting stronger. It often works well for stay-at-home parents and coworkers who need to get a workout in when it is convenient. For example, you might join a coworker for a workout during your lunch hour. Or maybe you are a parent who sees other parents at a sporting practice for your child; you can exercise together while you wait for the kids to finish. Choosing a reliable partner to train with increases the chance of you staying with your fitness program.

Another benefit to working out with a partner, especially when it comes to lifting weights, is safety. It is dangerous to lift heavy weights without someone there to spot you. Plus, a partner can provide some healthy competition while keeping each other safe. It is fun to visit with each other between sets; however, you do not want to "visit" too much and miss a challenging workout and its results. Actually, the best place to find a workout partner is at the gym, if that is where you are going to train together. Partnering up can help you try different exercises and move you forward.

Group Fitness

Group fitness works well for those who like some interaction with a group of people and may not want to participate solo with another person only. Some people like to combine social time with exercise, typically with like-minded people. Good examples are walkers, runners, and cyclists. It's a "we are all in this together" mentality when you are part of a fitness group, and it promotes a feeling of community. If you are feeling tired or need some encouragement, just look around you and the other members of the group can pull you through. If one person has to go out of town and miss class, there are others who will still show up.

The trick to working out with a group is finding a timeslot that works for your schedule. A group exercise program may or may not meet your specific needs. Evaluating your fitness results is important when working out within a group to make sure you are reaching your goals. It's important to have an instructor in a group setting who offers a variety of exercises and challenges. All movements can be modified for each person. People can pair off and do two-person exercises using medicine balls or resistance bands for a change of pace. Shared workouts can translate into better problem solving and teamwork in fitness and in life.

Are You A Couple?

When a couple schedules time to exercise or pursue a fitness activity together, it is a great way to have quality time together. If you're in a relationship, it is important to have balance. If you eat a decadent meal together, make a plan to work it off together. Working out together can be just as gratifying quality time as a Hulu or Netflix series.

Reaching your fitness goals is always more successful when the person(s) closest to you is on board —you can support each other. Working out with your partner during your workout can spill over into your relationship for a stronger bond and connection. Let's be honest, though — I have had some relationships where I could do almost anything with that partner but work out. If you are in a relationship where there is more bickering or criticism than training, it might sabotage your workout efforts.

Before you decide to train with your partner, take the time to discuss your individual and shared goals and make a rule of "no critics allowed" for at least your one-hour of exercise. Many couples find working out together builds trust, respect, and more attraction to each other. They rely on each other's strengths and it helps them feel good about themselves and as a couple. Flirting along the way and comments such as "nice biceps!" keeps you both connected in more ways than one.

Regardless, you decide whether you work out with your spouse, train with a workout partner or simply enjoy group fitness classes. The more people actively engaged in your health and fitness goals, the better. You have to know you're only competing with yourself and it's never going to be a lifetime thing if you aren't honest with yourself and learn to enjoy the process.

BUDGETING TIME AND MONEY

Time and money are things we all have to deal with on a daily basis, but how can you put a price on your health? Participating in health and fitness activities pays off dividends over and over again for years to come. Budgeting your time for exercise is one of the smartest things you can do for yourself. Schedule it. Work around your exercise program. Consider budgeting your time for exercise as a gift to yourself — an investment in you.

Investing in regular physical activity will save you money down the road by preventing illness and disease, which can occur when exercise is not a part of your life. You make an appointment to go to work every day or schedule time to get your hair done. You have to put yourself on your schedule. The same is true for your workouts.

FAKE IT TILL YOU MAKE IT

Read a biography or website online about a person and you will realize while most of it may be true, much of the information is embellished or exaggerated. A person's accomplishments, knowledge, and experience may be overstated or inflated, however many find it gets them to the next level in their career. "Fake it till you make it" works with fitness as well. As you continue to grow knowledgeable and experienced in your workouts and eating habits, it helps boost your confidence and reach your next level of fitness.

RAGS-TO-RICHES STORY

It was a long struggle for Suze Orman, who started out as a waitress and became one of television's most well-known financial gurus. She will admit she has had more failures than successes over the years, but she truly believes you learn so much from those failures and mistakes. Loss is a gift — though it may not feel like it at the time. Here is a perfect example of someone who faked it until she made it. She got real honest with herself, stood in her truth and that is when everything started to turn around for her.

To be honest, you are not really faking anything. It is normal to feel a little anxious about your next workout or about an exercise you have never done before, just as you may not have been able to imagine eating certain healthy foods that you've now incorporated into your new lifestyle. Faking it till you make it actually keeps you on your toes, and reaching your fitness goals gives you the confidence you deserve.

Theodore Roosevelt believed that "comparison is the thief of joy"; this is true and science has proved it — we need to stop making comparisons. Focus on your health, feeling better, having more energy, and losing weight (if that's one of your goals). Stop comparing yourself to the women and men in magazines who have been airbrushed to look "perfect."

Own the fact that you made yourself a priority and realized you needed to do something about your health and face your challenge. You are starting your journey by reading this book, getting prepared by cleaning out your cupboards of junk foodm and, if you stay completely honest with yourself about your health, you will gain confidence from both your success and failures along the way. Family and friends should support you as opposed to sabotaging your efforts.

By focusing on your strong points, continuing to perform the exercises you like to do (and those you don't) and making healthy meals, there is no doubt in my mind that you will develop your expertise on your health and wellness. You won't have to fake anything — you will simply be the best version of you. Be your own personal trainer.

HOW TO BUILD A HOME GYM ON A BUDGET

It may have occurred to you that if you had a gym at home, it would save you time and money when it comes to your fitness life. But what would it cost? What would it take? Where do you start? Of course, you do not want to buy a BowFlex machine and have it turn out to be utilized as a coat rack; however, the best time to buy fitness equipment is about a month or two after Christmas. The New Year's Resolutions are over and many companies offer sales online and in stores. Even if you have budgeted your time, you may find you still don't have the time to get to and from the gym.

Building a home gym costs less than you might think, but it is not for everyone. Some people cannot get motivated to exercise regularly without going outside the home to a gym. I know the days I don't want to do cardio I run to the gym and get a machine behind the fittest girl in the room as motivation. The biggest mistake many people make is spending a fortune on a fancy treadmill but never using it. When setting up your home gym, make sure the space is a refuge from all the other distractions going on in your home and personal life: kids, overflowing laundry, etc.

Dedicate a room with a door that you can close and not get interrupted. Invest in a stereo so you can play motivational music to exercise by as well as a mirror. This is not being vain; to lower your risk of injury, you need to make sure you watch your form and technique as you exercise. For some, investing in a high-quality mat that will easily fit in your living room or bedroom works well with a video to watch for doing yoga, Pilates or both. Maybe you can do your cardio work outside.

Home gyms do not have to be huge. However, simply buying a treadmill or bicycle is not enough. Cardiovascular exercises are not enough. A combination of resistance training and cardio is best for weight loss and overall fitness. Weight training tones muscle, adds definition, and is the best way to lose weight efficiently. Two or three sets of dumbbells or a set of adjustable ones work well and will allow you the option of doing a variety of exercises. Adjustable dumbbells with plates you can adjust easily are compact and a must for any home gym.

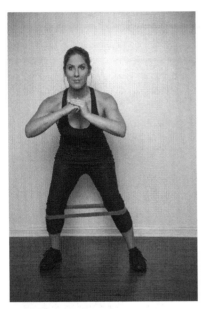
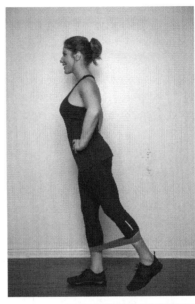

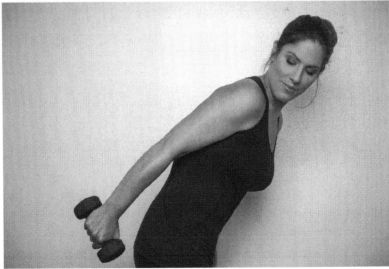

COMPARISON IS THE ROOT OF ALL EVIL

Comparing ourselves to others is quite normal. We do it with our homes, clothes, and jobs, and it seems to never end. But we can still be objective. Comparison can also have a positive impact on our daily lives — it can give us ideas for what we might want to shop or look for in the future.

However, there is a negative side to comparing ourselves to others, especially when aspirational images are everywhere we look: online, on billboards, and on television. We need to acknowledge the fact that we are all different shapes and sizes. Comparing yourself to others can be harmful if you find it alters how you view yourself or puts you in a bad mood. It can make you question your progress towards good health or weight loss, and that's not good. Be careful how you talk to yourself, because you are listening — especially now, as we are resetting.

The next time you find yourself scrolling through your Facebook page or the latest fashion magazine, ask yourself if they used lighting, different poses or body angles to make themselves look perfect in the picture. If you are struggling with comparing yourself to others, avoid magazines and social media for a little while. Remember, you have something to be proud of: you are focusing on improving your health. Bravo. The happiest people do not have to share every single thing about their lives. Learn something new.

IS YOUR BRAIN DESIGNED TO BE NEGATIVE?

For many years, scientists have been studying the brain and its impact on our beliefs about behavior and motivation that have a significant impact on us all. As humans, we have always been aware of and worked hard to avoid danger. In other words, people are hard-wired to be positive or negative, especially during difficult or dangerous times. Our desire to avoid negative experiences tends to outweigh our desire to seek out positive ones. Fear is a gift.

The negative perspective is often more infectious than the positive perspective. Our attitude is more heavily influenced by bad news than good news. In the English dictionary, there are more negative emotional words (62%) than positive ones (32%). When you detect negative experiences or start looking for bad news, it is quickly stored in our long-term memory.

Research shows that positive experiences have to be held in our awareness for more than 12 seconds in order to transfer them from our short-term to long-term memory. It seems odd, but Rick Hanson of *The Huffington Post* was quoted as saying, "The brain is like Velcro for negative experiences but Teflon for positive ones."

A recent study published in The Journal of Abnormal Psychology conducted by Jason Moser and his colleagues at Michigan State University showed that people have a hard time putting a positive spin on difficult situations, and actually make negative emotions worse even when they are asked to think positively. In fact, many people who are critical and say negative things, as opposed to giving praise, are often viewed as more intelligent.

Unless we occupy our brain with positive thoughts, worrying is our default position. We have to constantly strive to control our consciousness and direct our attention to activities that give us positive feedback and strengthen our sense of purpose and achievement. In other words, we can learn to keep our negative emotions in check by strengthening and intensifying our positive emotions.

Here are some suggestions to think about and apply to your daily life with yourself and others:

If there is a particular problem or situation you are dealing with in your life, particularly when it comes to your health and wellness, think about the problem in a different way using different strategies. For example, if you are someone who is struggling with sugar cravings, figure out meals consisting of quality protein and fiber which will keep you full and will help you not crave sugar.

Be conscious of people who may sabotage your efforts to lose weight. They may be close friends, family members, or even parents. Make it clear you are on a journey of weight loss or better health and you would appreciate their support.

When you drop a dress size or your weight loss shows on the scale, celebrate this positive event in your life with something other than food. For example, schedule a pedicure or massage, or get a new hairstyle to go with your new weight loss.

Avoid over-analyzing the situation of eating unhealthy or making poor food choices. Focus on what you can do right now, in this present moment, to be proactive in correcting the situation. For example, you might grill some chicken breasts or roast some vegetables for the week ahead to help you stay on track with your eating plan.

Focus on the small improvements in your health, and take the time to celebrate those. You might keep a jar in the kitchen and put a dollar in for every pound lost, good night's sleep, or successful workout where you were able to do one more push-up. Give yourself regular and frequent positive reinforcements for all of your hard work.

Remember: it takes five to ten positive events to counterbalance one negative event.

IMPORTANCE OF FITNESS SPONSORS

When you think about a fitness sponsor, you might dream of scoring all sorts of free products, appearing in or on the cover of magazines, or landing some huge sponsorship deal, perhaps with a supplement company. However, you do not need to put some huge deal together or win a fitness competition (though that never hurts). Most companies are more interested in your persona or someone who has a huge following. If people look up to you as a role model for fitness, for example, that translates into people trusting your judgment, making it easier for a company to build credibility and a strong customer base.

Social networking is an excellent way to build your followers and perhaps promote what you are doing. There is nothing better than having support online and sharing your experience with getting in shape. Perhaps you have a few favorite exercises, group fitness classes, or an exercise routine that really made a difference in your physique you would like to share with others who might be struggling with their weight loss. Create a website or write a blog so it makes it easier for people to reach you. Be a VERB. Be on social media for a bigger purpose. You never know where it might lead.

Sometimes sponsors are looking for those who are knowledgeable about their product line or they might be looking for someone who is not afraid to talk to people in stores or gyms. How you present yourself to the world, your personality, and attitude all have an impact when you show your true self. Many companies look for people who are comfortable with speaking about their product or how you were successful in your weight loss journey. It is up to you.

One of the best ways to get a sponsor for you or an event is to visit the company's website to get an idea of what they are all about or what they do. Many companies list careers available or offer an online application to be a member of their contracted athletes list. Learn all you can about the company before you contact them. Do some research on the company's demographics and company goals, how it all started and the brains behind the operation — be prepared. Think about what you are looking for in a sponsorship and what you want from a company. After talking with you, most companies will be able to tell how sincere you are or if you are just looking for the spotlight.

Most people who get sponsored do this because they are passionate about the health and fitness industry. Make the right relationships and build a foundation that can take you further than you ever dreamed. For example, if you are interested in a supplement company, you should be willing to work just to get free supplements. Very few people receive both money and supplements, especially if you are just starting out. Building a strong foundation will open up all sorts of doors.

It may take you getting involved with the customers or fans and really caring about what you do and what the company stands for. Give more than 100% of your time and effort. Learn all you can about the company and do what is needed. Be helpful. Sponsorship is an ongoing process translated from your personal life to official work and events. Keep in mind sponsorships are rare, but you should not lose hope or take rejection personally. Do what you love and work hard to make relationships with companies that do or sell what you believe in.

IMPORTANCE OF PROTEIN AND THE DIFFERENT TYPES

Protein is a very important macronutrient that repairs and maintains tissues including every organ, tissue, and cell in our bodies. Protein is made up of amino acids which are the building blocks of protein. The body needs twenty different amino acids. Eight of them are known as the essential amino acids, since they cannot be made by the body and must be obtained from food. The other twelve are made by the body and are known as non-essential amino acids.

Our bodies are constantly breaking down proteins and replacing them. In other words, the body does not store amino acids like it does fats and carbohydrates. The body needs a daily supply of amino acids to make new proteins. The protein in the food we eat is digested into amino acids that are used to replace the proteins in our body.

Different Types of Protein

A complete protein source is one that provides all of the essential amino acids. Complete proteins come from animal sources such as poultry, fish, eggs, meat and milk, including foods made from soy (tempeh and tofu). We should consume about 75% of our protein from high quality sources. An incomplete protein source is one low in one or more of the essential amino acids. Most plant proteins are incomplete proteins such as those found in nuts and legumes. Incomplete proteins can be combined to obtain protein of sufficient quality to be considered complete such as beans and rice.

Good sources of protein include:

- Poultry
- Chicken

- Lean meats
- Fish
- Eggs with egg whites
- Dry beans and peas
- Tofu and tempeh

A 3-ounce piece of meat contains about 21 grams of protein

1 cup of dry beans contains 16 grams of protein

The Role of Protein in the Body

Protein is important for many functions in the body. It is important for building, maintaining, and repairing body tissues. In addition to structural components such as muscles, bones, skin, organs, protein is a big part of hormones and enzymes that function to regulate body processes. Protein makes antibodies so we can fight disease. If you do not consume enough fat and carbohydrate, proteins can supply your body with plenty of energy.

You need about 8 grams of protein for every 20 pounds of body weight. That translates to about 46 grams of protein per day for women and 56 grams of protein for men.

Protein Needs for Older Adults

Current research and expert opinion, however, shows the RDA for protein of 0.8 grams per kilogram of body weight may not be adequate as we age. The current RDA was made based on research in young adults and does not promote optimal health or protect older adults from muscle loss and function with aging. Older adults need 1.2 grams of protein per kilogram of body weight or higher per day.

Additionally, an adequate amount of protein intake with each meal is important to promote protein anabolism or protein building. An intake of 25 to 30 grams of high-quality protein per meal is necessary for optimal muscle protein synthesis. Protein intakes at this level are particularly beneficial for older adults as a strategy to maintain muscle mass.

Protein has many important roles in our bodies and is part of every tissue, including our organs, muscles, and skin. You need to make sure you eat enough high-quality protein in your diet, especially as you age so your body has the amino acids it needs to function properly. Older adults may need more protein than current recommendations to help optimize their health and protect their lean muscle mass.

KEEP YOUR CULTURE – BUT UPDATE YOUR COOKING

Whatever your culture or background, you can still enjoy your favorite foods by updating your cooking methods and ingredients. A healthy diet, regardless of your culture, can still focus on lean protein sources, whole grains, fresh fruits and vegetables with moderate amounts of dairy products such as Greek yogurt. For example, whole-grain foods provide a huge opportunity to make ethnic choices healthier: such as whole-grain pasta, brown rice, couscous, barley, or bulgur wheat. High-fiber foods help support a healthy digestive system.

Spend some time in your ethnic cookbooks or search online for ethnic recipes. When you start reading the ingredients, find alternatives for healthier options. For example, instead of using all butter, use olive oil. Many ethnic cooking styles use familiar ingredients with different mixes of spices and herbs. Making a few simple changes can allow you to still enjoy your favorite ethnic dish with less fat, salt, and sugar. Add more vegetables to a dish or find ways to lower the fat and increase the fiber and other nutrients.

Tips and Strategies For Eating Healthy Ethnic Foods

Many traditional dishes can be high in calories, fat and sodium. Appetizers are an excellent way to enjoy some ethnic foods with less fat and calories. Many Latino dishes use rice, beans, and tortillas, all of which are high in carbohydrates. However, there are plenty of tricks to allow you to still prepare these foods that are more nutritious, flavorful and authentic. Black bean tacos or tacos made with ground turkey help reduce the fat content. Here are some examples:

Healthy Mexican

Choose options that include lean poultry, fresh seafood and beans as your protein source. Add guacamole for some good fat and experiment with different salsas for added flavor. Measure out one serving of whole-grain chips with some salsa — this way you can still enjoy your favorite food without going overboard.

Healthy Italian

Italian is one of my favorite ethnic foods, and you can still enjoy it using healthier options. For example, use whole-grain pasta and ground turkey meat for spaghetti. Look for a tool, like a spiralizer, that allows you to create noodles with zucchini, and toss with olive oil, garlic, and Italian herbs. Believe me… it is delicious.

Whenever you create an ethnic meal, use a dinner plate for the salad and vegetable portion. Use a salad plate for the protein source and whole grains.

USE HEALTHY COOKING METHODS

Regardless of your favorite ethnic meal, it is a great time to fire up the grill to cook your fish, vegetables and chicken outdoors. Of course, baking, steaming, and broiling will reduce the amount of fat you use when cooking your favorite ethnic food. Also, go easy with the cheese, as it is high in fat and sodium. In place of sour cream, use plain Greek yogurt in recipes.

Regardless of your choice of ethnic foods, it is possible to enjoy healthier versions that will not derail your weight loss efforts. Bellisimo!

CLIENT STORY: GWEN

My father trained people throughout the 1980s in between filmmaking. I remember a story about one of his clients that still resonates with me to this day. This story made me not only sad when I was a little girl, but also had me really start to think deeper about why people behave like they do.

My father took on a woman named "Gwen" to train. Gwen was in her 60s and weighed well over 350 pounds. She was 5'3", soft-spoken, and never married. Gwen came to Lou to find out how to train properly and get help with her diet and nutrition. Gwen and Lou trained for months together. Every week, Gwen would come to the gym on time and meet him outside at the entrance. Though Gwen worked hard and was disciplined in the gym, she wasn't losing any weight. When confronted, Gwen swore up and down that she was following Lou's nutritional advice and was cracking down on her heavy fat and sugar intake.

One morning, around 9:10 a.m., and there was no sign of Gwen. It was so unlike Gwen to be even 5 minutes late for a workout, so Lou went to look for Gwen's car. As Lou approached Gwen's car, he noticed Gwen still in it. Lou knocked on the window and startled Gwen who seemed to be lost in her own world. When Gwen opened the door, he could see an empty box of doughnuts and numerous bags of fast food wrappers. The look Gwen gave Lou broke his heart. He said it was the look of a child being told that their favorite goldfish had died and they were to blame.

Gwen immediately broke down but instead of running away like she wanted to, and was used to doing in her life, agreed to sit and talk with Lou in private. Gwen was an only child to Orthodox Jewish parents. Her mother was supportive and loving to her, but her father, who had survived the concentration camps, was cold and strict. Gwen was raised with the philosophy (by her father) that children were to be "seen and not heard." She remembers beatings from her father if her grades were not high and, especially, if she didn't eat every bite on her plate. Because her father worked hard to provide to put food on the table, hungry or not, Gwen had to eat or she would be beaten.

Gwen started to drastically add on weight when she was 8 years old. She would eat everything on her plate and then sneak to her room and find her hidden stash of sweets and eat them as well. Instead of enjoying the sweets like she once did, over time, she mainly used them to emotionally push down the depression, loneliness, and anxiety she felt living in isolation in her home.

Gwen compared her emotional eating to a drug habit. Food was her only friend and her escape mechanism. Like a drug, overeating numbed her sadness at the moment; all her feelings triggering her behavior were still there. After the sugar high, Gwen would feel worse than she did before. Gwen constantly felt powerless and beat herself up for not having more willpower; this cycle went on for over five decades. Her secrets led her into isolation and missing out on many aspects of life because her real internal issues were never addressed.

EXCUSE #5:
I WILL START ON MONDAY

After following your new strategies for a month, you may have "failed" to stick to your best eating plan or skipped a workout or a day of journaling at least once, if not many times. We are human. This is also realistically the point where you might start to become "bored" with the discipline required and aren't seeing your body lean out as fast as you would like. This chapter offers strategies for minimizing the damage and keeping on track by exploring a version of the popular excuse "I will start Monday."

You will be guided through specific cardio and strength training "upgrades" this week, as well as challenged to begin making even healthier choices regarding gluten within the parameters of your food plan. You will also be asked to review your journal and repeat the fitness assessment exercises, assess your progress and change in different areas to create new strategies for staying motivated and moving toward your goals.

WHAT DOES IT MEAN TO FAIL?

What you may not realize is when you put your all into a new healthy eating plan, you may fail at some point because you are allowing the "eating plan" to take control. In my opinion, failure is when you give up your power in life. We all get knocked down at times and fail at times, but it is not real failure unless you do not choose to get back up again. You may think to yourself, "why should I be motivated to try again?" especially when you may not know how you fell down in the first place.

LET'S LOOK AT SOME FAD DIETS

The Banting Diet From 1863

Years before the Atkins diet came around, William Banting created a diet book after trying to lose weight for over 20 years. He had tried every fad diet the experts of that day recommended, but nothing worked. In fact, he continued to gain weight and could no longer tie his shoelaces. Plus, he had hearing problems. The ear, nose, and throat doctor placed him on an eating plan that cut out bread, milk, sugar, beer and potatoes and he lost a pound a week. As a result, his hearing came back, eyesight improved and he created a more active lifestyle. The word of his strategy spread and the word "bant" became a verb known as "banting", meaning losing weight.

Do You Remember The Grapefruit Diet?

It became a huge fad in the 1980s and you may have heard it is making a comeback. In addition to eating grapefruit, you are advised to eat hard-boiled eggs and drink black coffee. You might lose weight on this 800-calorie-per-day, unhealthy eating plan, but it is certainly not the way to lead a balanced, healthy lifestyle. You can certainly enjoy a grapefruit as part of your eating plan for fruits and vegetables, but long-lasting weight loss needs consistency with healthy foods and beverages that leave you feeling full and satisfied.

The Cabbage Soup Diet

In the 1950s, the cabbage soup diet became all the rage, promising weight loss of 10 pounds in one week. There are many versions of the diet; however, most of the weight loss is water and precious muscle tissue, not body fat. Common complaints include flatulence and fatigue or lightheadedness due to a lack of calories and protein. This is definitely not the way to go to lose weight and keep it off. Avoid the cabbage soup diet altogether. It lacks proper nutrition, can cause dizziness and flatulence, and is not sustainable.

Weight Watchers

Housewife Jean Nidetch, who described herself as "overweight and obsessed with cookies," started Weight Watchers. The program is based on a point system assigning specific points to each food item based on the amount of calories, fat and fiber. Exercise is encouraged and allows you to earn extra points. I am not a fan of the point system because you could be allowed 85 points and eat them all by noon. Then what do you do? While Weight Watchers has changed over the years and now encourages eating whole, unprocessed foods, they still used products with preservatives, point counting instead of nutrient counting and the focus is predominantly on the scale only to measure success.

Nutrisystem

The company's mission statement is to "provide a weight loss program based on quality foods and a nutritionally balanced meal plan." We feel the same with our program, "Incredibly FIT" by Ferrigno FIT.

In 2001 I was really interested in food and diets, and decided to join the 28-day $299 program to see if their prepackaged meals were in fact quality food. I was in college and busy. I gave up my school meal plan for a month. When I found out I was going to be told what to eat with no emphasis on grocery shopping and nutritional education, I was disappointed. Then, when I tasted the prepackaged meals, I was *done*.

Depending on the person, the daily caloric allowance varies from 1,200 to 1,500 calories. I believe in diet, but pushing yourself to exercise as well. I am active so I took the 1,400-calorie option. I was delivered 18 ready-to-go foods and 10 days' worth of frozen food. I was given 3 meals and 2 snacks a day. After my first day I was shocked to find out the average customer sticks with it 9.5 weeks (66.5 days); this interested me because I believe in 66 days you can break habits, with the right education and foundation.

When people are giving up at 66.5 days with Nutrisystem, my clients are just beginning to break the next habit. The food ratio was 55% carbs, 25% protein and 20% fat. With each month you get a call allowance to get extra advice from Nutrisystem employees; whether the people on the other end were credentialed or not, I couldn't tell. I was told many things I don't agree with, but what set me off was being told diet soda was okay — that's a big NO in my opinion (I will explain later in the book) — and I did not learn much about food because my meals were already provided. In this book, you will see I encourage you to steer clear from preservatives and sodium.

Nutrisystem takes pride in their meals being low-calorie and low-fat. The meals may be, but in my opinion they taste awful, are filled with sodium and left me feeling constantly hungry and disappointed. I hated how alienated I felt on their program. At dinner parties I would warm up prepackaged meals that were assigned to me while my friends were going with what they were craving and making theirs fresh. As soon as I began losing a few pounds, I was bored and so frustrated by hanger (hungry anger) that I ditched the program entirely.

Nutrisystem recently hired celebrity chefs to make the meals more tolerable;

with "Incredibly FIT" by Ferrigno FIT, you become your own personal chef and trainer. I felt better off the Nutrisystem program and was so thankful when I started making my meals myself. In my book they got a 2/5.

Pros:
- The macronutrients ratio
- Support
- Community

Cons:
- The prepackaged meals
- Preservatives
- Lack of education
- Taste

Slim-Fast

It was 1977 — oh, Slim-Fast. This non-refrigerated chocolate drink — meal replacement — should be called "Slim-More-sugar-than-a-Hershey-bar"; the original Slim-Fast has 34 grams of sugar, while a Hershey bar has 24. I love to eat and have never been the type of girl who fasted or juiced. There are many different reasons, but a big one is I like to eat my food.

I did the old school Slim-Fast routine: a shake for breakfast, 2 Slim-Fast bars as a snack, another shake for lunch, and a 500-calorie dinner of my choosing. They advertise that each serving contains between 180 and 190 calories and provides about one-third of your daily recommended intake for vitamins and minerals. There are four different flavors: chocolate, vanilla, strawberry and cappuccino. I was over it by the second day.

Again, I went old-school with my shakes and didn't opt for the sweetened flavored ones. I was constantly hungry; I chewed on ice to feel satisfied after the shake, and hated the taste. I should have loved it because of the sugar in it — but I also knew that was the reason I was constantly hungry. With the lack of education, support and guidance, I am shocked that this fad is still around. The ingredients contain a ton of controversial ingredients, but when I read about it having Acesulfame-K… it was over. Acesulfame-K is a potassium salt that contains methylene choloride, a carcinogen. When exposed to this carcinogen long-term, it's been known to cause headaches, impaired mood, eyesight, nausea, liver, and kidney issues.

If you can't pronounce or have an idea of what an ingredient is on the label, you shouldn't take it. In this book, you will see how you can get your minerals and nutrients from fresh, natural and balanced food/vitamins without carcinogens and side effects. Slim-FAT, you get a 1/5… and I am being nice.

Pros:

- Fast weight loss
- Minerals and Vitamins

Cons:

- Ingredients
- Hunger
- Lack of Education
- Taste
- Preservatives

The New Beverly Hills Diet

The New Beverly Hills Diet Program is based on and designed around the best-selling 1981 book *The Beverly Hills Diet* written by actress Judy Mazel.

The 35-day diet is a food combination encouraging the dieter to be conscious about their food, eating times, and eating combos. Mazel's philosophy with weight loss and weight gain have to do less with how much you eat and more about the times you eat and food combinations. Her theory is based on the fact that when some foods are eaten together, it leads to poor digestion and eventually obesity. Mazel suggests having fat is simply a symptom of poor digestion and when your body is digesting food properly, you will lose body fat.

On the first day of the diet, I was instructed to eat pineapple, corn on the cob, and a salad made of lettuce, tomatoes, and onions with "Mazel dressing." Mazel emphasizes her dressing constantly and I felt pressured to buy it, feeling like I wouldn't succeed at the program if I didn't. That irked me and always does. I would have been better with simple balsamic vinegar.

Because I started with the pineapple I could eat as much pineapple as I wanted, but when I wanted to move on to eating my corn on the cob I couldn't go back and eat more pineapple. It was the same progression plan with the salad. When I was in salad land, both corn on the cob and pineapple are no longer allowed. She encourages her dieters to take time between each new food group.

The New Beverly Hills Diet promises the dieters if they follow their theory they will lose up to 25 pounds in 35 days. I lost 5 but didn't stick with it. Mazel based her program off her personal 72-pound weight-loss journey, not from a nutritional degree or any professional education. Though a wide variety of food is an option, you are allowed to eat carbohydrates only with other carbohydrates, proteins only with other proteins, and fruit alone.

I found this program hard to manage and completely different from the way I work; what's meat without a potato? My digestion was on point, but the portion control concept and maintenance plan after the 35 days was non-existent. There is no calorie restriction with the plan, which is confusing once you graduate and it has no emphasis on exercise whatsoever.

Pros:

- Variety of foods
- Digestion education

Cons:

- No exercise guidance
- Hard to manage long-term
- No portion control education
- No maintenance plan
- Mazel is not a trusted expert

Atkins Diet

Dr. Atkins published the Dr. Atkins Diet Revolution in the 1970s and the protein craze began the world's misguided hatred for carbohydrates. Carbohydrates' reputation has never quite recovered from this diet fad, which had a huge comeback in 1994.

Robert Atkins, MD wrote the book Dr. Atkins' Diet Revolution in 1972. The theory is that when you drastically cut back on carbs, your body turns to your fat stores for fuel. The result is you burn body fat, releasing a by-product called ketones you'll use for energy. That made sense to me. Let's make sure you understand the different terminology:

Saturated Fats — Saturated fats are natural and come from animal fat products. You can find it in butter, lard, and fatty meats. The American Heart Association suggests for a 2,000-calorie diet and no more than 120 of them should come from saturated fats, suggesting 13 grams of saturated fat a day.

Trans Fats (partially hydrogenated oils) — These fats are produced naturally in meat, but where you find them the most is in shelved foods like cookies, crackers and breads. Trans fat is a big staple in the fast food community. Trans fat is artificial and began when companies were trying to find a cheap alternative to butter that also acted as a preservative. Considering how unnatural it is, trans fat is worse than any saturated fat in your diet.

Simple Carbohydrates — Simple carbohydrates are sugar. They are digested quickly and spike your energy level at a fast speed. They hit you quick and wear off fast. Examples of these simple sugars include:

1. Table Sugar
2. Corn Syrup
3. Soda
4. Candy

Complex Carbohydrates — Your go-to carbs should be complex carbohydrates. Unlike simple carbs, these carbohydrates are rich in fiber and leave you satisfied longer. They are rich in vitamins and minerals and include:

1. Oatmeal
2. Starchy vegetables (potatoes, corn)
3. Green vegetables
4. Beans
5. Lentils
6. Whole grains

Atkins is not a perfect diet and the concept could be considered flawed, but it far surpassed the diets consisting of trans fat and simple carbs. If done correctly, it can kick some bad food habits/and or addictions. It brings awareness to the difference between quality and quantity; teaching me about saturated fat, protein choices, and why carbs make you hungry. Though I wasn't hungry, I was needy for carbs, and, though I knew I couldn't sustain Atkins as a lifestyle, it was the healthier and fresher option for me.

Pros:

- Fresh food approach
- Not constantly hungry
- Professional opinion
- Does not promote trans fat
- Lack of sugar helped my overall mood

Cons:

- Missed carbs
- Tired in the beginning
- Breath stank

The South Beach Diet

Considered the more moderate version of Atkins, Miami's Dr. Arthur Agatston added fuel to the low-carb craze by publishing "The South Beach Diet." Unlike the Atkins diet, Agatston believes in swapping saturated fats for unsaturated ones and supports eating "I Can't Believe It's Not Butter." Agatston, a leading cardiologist, created this program for his heart patients. The diet has three phases, but if you have less than 10 pounds to lose, you can start the program with phase 2.

His motto is that this diet is not a low fat or low-carb diet, but rather teaches you how to eat the right carbs and fats. He promotes eating three meals a day, two snacks, and a high-protein dessert (chocolate mousse). I like that he doesn't have an end date with this diet, and like my 66-day program, once the phases are done, he encourages you to do it again until you hit your weight loss goal.

He limits saturated fats but mentions "I Can't Believe It's Not Butter" is fine to use. However, that is fake food and a *huge* no-no in my eyes. The book claims you can lose 8-13 pounds the first two weeks and 1-2 pounds each following week. Most weight loss, he claims, will come from your stomach. I can understand that because by having to restrict carbohydrates in the first two weeks, it will help with your digestive system, leaving you feeling less bloated. Each phase becomes less restrictive. He refers back to the Glycemic Index often, but in my opinion, doesn't give the best guidance on how to use it.

When I read that he believed 20 minutes of exercise a day is enough I was extremely disappointed. Instead of having the vision that his book is for everyone, I began to believe it was for people already in shape, and was just looking to get in bikini-ready shape to walk along the Atlantic Ocean in Miami.

Pros:

- Limiting saturated fats
- Teaches you how to eat real food
- Affordable and online tools available
- Expert advice
- Promotes lower carbs and higher protein
- Teaches you how to change your eating habits

Cons:

- Lack of exercise advice
- Not enough detail about the Glycemic Index
- First phase restricts carbs and can leave you feeling nauseous, tired, and dizzy

When we talk about the fad diets, though they update them and add new features, they will never be 100% successful if they don't talk about mental well-being with the program. Weight Watchers has now started to do this but still offers their horrible high-sodium meals. Their new program is called "Beyond the Scale" and was developed in response to changing science about nutrition. In other words, weight is not the only focus of the Weight Watchers program. The points have changed with a new points program called Smart Points.

Weight Watchers now looks at the type of fat in a particular food. Their new formula looks at saturated fat more heavily. Lean protein sources are encouraged. Fruits and vegetables still have zero points. The daily and weekly allotments have changed and are based on the person's resting metabolic rate. Plus, exercise was not always a part of the program; now, each member has an exercise goal. Members are encouraged to do non-food related activities that make them feel good about themselves. At least there have been some improvements in their program.

DITCHING THE WILLPOWER AND TAKING BACK YOUR CONTROL

Besides insulin, when you eat something sweet your brain releases dopamine, which turns on your brain's pleasure center making you feel pleasure like you would during sex. Dopamine, which is responsible for energy, memory, and focus, has receptors all over our brain and when triggered enough by sweets as well as fats leads to increased amounts of dopamine causing brain behavior similar to that of an addict. The more sugar or drugs you take, the higher your tolerance, the more you crave it, and the more it leaves you feeling desperate and out of control. The appetite-regulating hormone leptin is also released, whose job is to tell your brain you are "full" once a certain amount of calories have been consumed.

When you consume something that tastes sweet but doesn't have any calories, your brain's reward center still gets alerted by the sweet taste. The problem is, unlike sugar, there's nothing to turn it off, since the calories never arrive.

Artificial sweeteners basically trick your body into thinking it's going take in sugar — but when the sugar doesn't come, your body begins to crave sweets, which leads to eating more. The FDA has approved 5 artificial sweeteners that all taste much sweeter than table sugar:

- **Aspartame:** Equal and NutraSweet is 180 times sweeter than sugar

- **Acesulfame-K:** Sweet One is 200 times sweeter than sugar

- **Saccharin:** Sweet N' Low and Necta Sweet is 300 times sweeter than sugar

- **Sucralose:** Splenda is 600 times sweeter than sugar
- **Neotame:** Newest sweetener to be FDA approved and is 7,000 to 13,000 sweeter than sugar

Over the last 40 years there have been countless studies about the effects sweeteners have on your overall health. Some say they help you, but most say they're harmful and others believe they do cause obesity, cardiovascular diseases, and even cancer. There is no consistent proof to most of these assertions, but people continue to consume these chemicals because they are approved by the FDA and available on market shelves all around the world. Let's make one HUGE misconception clear:

The FDA does not hire scientists to independently study a product for review. The companies fund the studies and the FDA is simply in charge of evaluating them. This leaves a lot of room for shadiness.

Sucralose is allowed to call their products "natural" because it is derived from sugar, but in no way is a product processed in a factory and filled with chemicals "natural." Agave is heavily processed and is almost 90% fructose. Don't be misled; there is nothing healthy about agave. According to the Market Research Report (2004), artificial sweeteners are added to about 6,000 different beverages, snacks, and food products.

In 1879, a chemistry research assistant, Constantine Fahlberg, accidentally discovered saccharin, making it the first artificial sweetener. Saccharin became popular after World War I and II when sugar was limited due to rationing. After the World Wars, saccharin's popularity only grew and it became a staple at restaurants and in many food products. The FDA banned cyclamate, a short-lived artificial sweetener, in 1969 because of its carcinogenic potentials, and started to hone in on all artificial sweeteners, making an attempt to ban saccharin in 1977. But because of popular demand, Congress extended the ban seven times to allow more test research to be done.

In 1965, James Schlatter, a chemist at G.D. Searle & Company also accidentally discovered a sugar substitute while testing an anti-ulcer drug, aspartame. Unlike saccharin, the FDA was not as kind to aspartame, the chemical used in Equal and NutraSweet products, triggering the first criminal investigation of a manufacturer in 1977. In 1980, the FDA Board of Inquiry banned aspartame based on the opinions of three independent scientists, after extensive research all agreed it "might induce brain tumors."

Donald Rumsfeld, American politician and businessman, was CEO of G.D. Searle & Co. during the time of the ban. In January of 1981 Rumsfeld addressed a sales meeting stating he was going to "call in his markers" and push hard to get aspartame approved. That same month President Reagan, an old friend of Rumsfeld, became the 40th President of the United States.

Rumsfeld became part of Regan's transition team and picked out personally Dr. Arthur Hull Hays Jr. to be the new FDA Director. A few months later Hayes picked a five-person Scientific Commission to go over the claims on aspartame. In a 3-2 vote the panel agreed aspartame was unsafe and decided to keep the ban on the sweetener.

Hays, having no experience with food additives, deadlocked the vote and then broke the tie to legalize it when he became the sixth member of the commission. In July, ignoring the studies showing that aspartame sickened and killed thousands of lab animals, Hayes approved aspartame in dry goods. In 1983, he approved aspartame in carbonated drinks right before he decided to resign due to accusations that he was accepting corporate gifts for political favors. Rumsfeld got exactly what he wanted when he received a 12-million dollar bonus when Searle was bought for 2.7 billion dollars by Monsanto in 1985.

WHAT COMPANIES DO TO MAKE UNHEALTHY FOODS LOOK SEXY

You can make great-tasting food without trying to fool people. There is no such thing as unhealthy foods, just unhealthy eating habits. The food industry needs to go back and read the USDA guidelines from the 1980s. The first two guidelines include eating a variety of foods and maintaining a healthy body weight. You can eat potato chips, or chocolate, or a prime rib of beef... just don't do it too often, and don't eat so much that you gain weight. It really is that simple.

The problem is that the simple advice first given by USDA is just not sexy enough. We need pyramids, pictures of plates, and stars on our food packages. Let's be honest, you can't just go on talk shows and say, "Eat sensibly." You need a gimmick. Otherwise, the message of the food industry could be "We make safe, delicious and inexpensive foods that, when eaten in moderation, are good for your body and mind."

There are many reasons why Americans have a love affair with unhealthy foods, snacks, and beverages. Those of you who can sit down in front of the television and polish off an entire bag of cookies or chips are proving exactly what the product was designed to do — be addictive. Drive by your local fast food restaurant and you can smell the overpowering scent of "something is cooking in the oven" or "cooking on the grill" that can entice the most discriminating eater. In the war of the food dollar, all tactics are feasible to manipulate how a food looks, smells and tastes in the mouth and nothing is left to chance.

There are food scientists and technologies using devices and ingredients to create food that promotes the perfect, creaminess, contract, crunch and blends flavors to lubricate mouthfuls so people eat faster. Plus, the actual time it takes to chew food has shrunk. In the past 50 years, we used to have foods we chewed at least 15 to 30 times before swallowing. Today, most foods only need to be chewed 12 times so you can get another hit of pleasure just a bit faster.

Add salt, sugar, and fat to the mix and you have hyper-palatable, hyper-rewarding, well-designed foods that drive our taste buds crazy and can literally override the brain's signal designed to tell us when to stop eating. Here are some foods that are deliberately designed to lure you in — hook, line, and sinker:

Soft Drinks — In addition to their caffeine, many people find soft drinks to be addictive and that is no accident. They contain malic, citric, and tartaric acids kept afloat with an additive known as brominated vegetable oil (BVO). Many soft drink companies are starting to drop this ingredient because it is also a flame retardant. However, you need to know that soft drinks are very addictive.

Cured Meats — Most people love bacon. However, sodium nitrite takes the credit for that yummy flavor. Sodium nitrites can also be found in hot dogs, sausages, ham, pastrami and salami. Nitrites also lengthen the shelf life of the product, gives the great color and pleasing taste everyone loves. The problem is, during the cooking process the nitrites combine with other chemicals and form carcinogens, something you want to avoid. Limit your intake.

Popcorn In The Microwave — Walk into any office that has a microwave oven and you know immediately if someone microwaved some popcorn. It can be almost impossible to resist the smell of butter flavoring chemicals like pentanedione and diacetyl filling the air from the heating process. In fact, there have been lawsuits brought about from "popcorn lung," a potentially fatal respiratory disease caused by constrictive bronchiolitis obliterans. The flow of air in the smallest airways of the lung become scarred and constricted, restricting movement of air. Resist microwave popcorn and make your own at home, on the stovetop, the old-fashioned way.

Baked, Fried, And Toasted Foods — Those toasted crisp breads, potato chips, salty roasted snacks, and even french fries are cooked at high temperatures to produce a golden brown surface that make them irresistible. Unfortunately, this process produces a cancer-causing chemical, acrylamide, that we should also resist. The other issue is when a food melts down quickly, your brain thinks there are no calories in it and you keep eating more and more. Add a coating of sugar, salt, and fat to the mix, and glucose levels go through the roof, making you crave more of the same.

Fast Food — Is established and based on addictions and cravings. Hence, you can always find a drive-thru window open that makes it quick and convenient to indulge in your favorite dish or entrée. If you are a fan of those nuggets of chicken though, I have some bad news. They are made with an anti-foaming agent called dimethylpolysiloxane, the same chemical used to make yoga mats and propylene glycol, an anti-freeze ingredient, plus an autolyzed yeast extract that enhances those cravings.

The next time you have cravings for fatty, salty, or sweet foods that can be hard to resist, know those foods are full of artificial flavorings, preservatives, and chemicals are designed to feed those cravings even more. Think twice before heading for a drive-thru and always keep healthy, whole-food ingredient snacks with you in your purse or car to can stop those cravings in a healthy way.

CREATING MINDFUL THINKING AND AWARENESS

Besides diet and exercise, it is important to be aware of your thoughts, feelings, and surroundings. Mindful eating means paying close attention to your body's hunger cues and learning to savor your food, as opposed to eating a hamburger while driving on the freeway. Mindfulness gets at the underlying causes of overeating, such as stress, cravings, or emotional eating that can be hard to defeat.

Ignoring any underlying dysfunctional relationship to food does not work. Trying to control eating through limit-setting or avoidance and thinking all you need is "willpower" is a myth. When eating plans go awry, many give up and binge or eat something unhealthy. However, from a more mindful perspective you can choose to eat mindfully any time of day, even after you have "blown it."

When you take the time to savor your food instead of avoiding it, you will not feel deprived. Take the guilt out of enjoying food and honor your healthy food preferences. Become your own "inner gourmand" and make better choices. If you really want a piece of cake, take a bite or two, then ask yourself, "Do I really want more?" *The Reset Plan* is not about dieting; it is about a lifestyle change that involves not fighting food anymore. You can do it. Practice mindful eating.

THE IMPORTANCE OF MEDITATION

Meditation reduces stress better than anything else you can do. It allows you to rest both mentally and physically and has a direct effect on your entire nervous system by reducing your body's production of stress hormones like cortisol. Plus, meditation helps increase the production of mood-enhancing chemicals like serotonin. Meditation improves your health by:

- Strengthening your immune system
- Reducing blood pressure
- Lowering cholesterol
- Supportting the healing process
- Improving sleep
- Slows down the aging process by reducing the body's production of free radicals
- Reduces anxiety

Meditation is a powerful tool that will help you in so many ways with your weight loss goals. However, you do not need to have any condition to reap the benefits from practicing meditation. In general, people who meditate are less stressed, sleep better, have a more positive outlook on life, and are happier.

MAKE IT EASY: UNDERSTANDING YOUR MEAL PLAN AND MEAL PREP

Are you feeling overwhelmed about your meal plan and preparation? Would you like to be more organized? Are you ready to quit already? You can do it. First and foremost, do not try to do it all today. Start slow and build on what you are comfortable with preparing. Take healthy recipes you prepare often and store them in the freezer or refrigerator. Think about what recipes would make it easier to prepare ahead of time.

For example, if dinnertime is stressful for you, invest in a slow cooker and place all the ingredients into it in the morning when you have more time. If you are someone who is always running to the vending machine at work for a snack, put together some vegetable packs with bags of almonds or hummus. Food preparation can be anything that makes it easier to create healthy meals throughout the week. The littlest bit of food preparation makes all the difference.

There are always going to be days when time is limited. Make the most of your time and prep whenever it suits you. There is no right or wrong way to prep food. It comes down to committing to getting it done and must be sustainable to fit into your lifestyle. Maybe you find it easy to boil a dozen eggs to keep in the refrigerator for the week or make salads for the next day's lunch the night before.

Give yourself some time to reap the rewards and make it a part of your new routine. Experience the benefits of forming new habits. It really does take three weeks to form a habit that works for you. You may have to make adjustments along the way but it is so worth it. It makes all the difference when you open up your refrigerator and find ready-to-eat snacks and healthy food for quick meals.

DETOXING – HOW IT FITS DURING & AFTER *THE RESET PLAN*

The word "toxin" comes to us from the Greek word *toxikon*, which means poison. Today, we refer to toxins as substances foreign to the human body that will eventually cause it harm or disease. It's very easy for your body to be overloaded with unhealthy toxins, as they're all around us. They're in the air we breathe, the food we eat, and the water we drink. Having a surplus of toxins in the body can lead to a host of health issues such as weight gain, fatigue, joint pain, and they can even effect the way your body functions on daily basis.

Your body is armed to defend toxins with natural detoxification systems to prevent their buildup. These include the liver, colon, kidneys, lungs, and skin. However, it's very easy for one of these channels to be impaired or overloaded with toxins. When this occurs, the body begins to accumulate toxins and ill health can result.

When your body is overwhelmed, there is an answer. To combat harmful toxins you can go through "cleanse" or "detox." Simply put, a cleanse or detox refers to the action of decreasing the body's toxic burden. This is achieved by controlling what you're putting in your body. Methods such as fasting, eating specific foods that promote detoxification, abstaining from foods that increase toxic load, and incorporating herbs or concoctions that promote toxic elimination are all great approaches to resetting your body's toxic load.

Did you know that we have been purifying our bodies through fasting, medicinal herbs and other means for thousands of years? In fact, there are written Chinese herbal prescriptions dating all the way back to 2700 BC. It's no wonder that you can open any health magazine and see nothing-but-juice cleanses, lemon water fasts, or even apple cider cleanses. It seems that "cleanses" and "detoxes" are just buzzwords in the health community. A lot of these buzzword cleanses and detoxes can be too steep of a gradient for many people and can result in feeling very ill as the toxic load is dumped faster than their body is able to process it.

However, that's not always the case. When you choose a cleanse/detox that is developed to gently assist the body's existing detoxification mechanisms, you can have great results that provide support rather than overwhelming your system. Unfortunately, most cleanses and detoxes on the market rely on marketing hype rather than science, which leads to poor results and massive confusion.

Choosing a high quality, science-based cleanse/detox can help rid the toxins while providing your body with what it craves to feel renewed, revitalized, and recharged. You'll not only be detoxifying your body and liver, but you may even see weight loss, curbed sugar cravings, and an increase in your energy levels.

I launched *The Reset Cleanse* to help me get back on track when I had a bad week or two with my eating choices during and after *The Reset Plan*. Life happens, especially around the holidays, but instead of giving up altogether I use our protein cleanse a few times a year to get back on track with my diet and goals. I took all the knowledge of what I had been working towards with the program and incorporated it with the cleanse. Besides myself I found it worked great with my clients. If you feel you are at the stage in *The Reset Plan* and you want to try the cleanse, to switch things up, you may be ready. Also, toxins do accumulate over time, so I suggest cleansing at least twice a year to make sure you're purging your body of anything that has over accumulated, which is inevitable to some extent. To learn more about the cleanse that I developed, look over all the information at **FerrignoFIT.com**.

SEROTONIN AND THE BRAIN

Serotonin is produced in the brain and intestines. In fact, most of your body's serotonin can be found in the gastrointestinal (GI) tract. It is also found in the central nervous system and blood platelets. It plays a major role in influencing a variety of psychological and bodily functions. Serotonin used inside the brain must be produced within it because it cannot cross the blood-brain barrier. Serotonin relays signals between the nerve cells, regulating their intensity as a neurotransmitter. Serotonin influences both indirectly and directly the majority of brains cells that affect:

- Mood
- Bowel function
- Blood clotting
- Sexual functioning
- Nausea
- Bone density

You can increase serotonin levels naturally through the following ways:

- Consume chickpeas or hummus – these are rich in tryptophan, the key component of serotonin
- Alterations in thought
- Light therapy – used as a treatment for Seasonal Affective Disorder (SAD)
- Regular exercise – has an antidepressant effect
- Diet – improves mood and cognition

BENEFITS OF GOAL-SETTING: LOCAL FITNESS EVENTS

Even the most disciplined person needs a little motivation, and there is nothing better than having an event or goal to aim for in the near future. Instead of being on autopilot by going to the gym every day and getting on the treadmill, you might want to consider the following:

- Walking or running a 5K for a charity
- Sign up for a mountain bike race
- Train for a bodybuilding or fitness contest

Whatever it is, participating in a fitness event can help prevent life getting in the way, or slipping on nutrition habits or simply doing an exercise that feels good. Having a goal can take you out of your comfort zone. Goals provide direction, and help channel your efforts in making the right decisions. They create motivation and help close the gap between where you are now and where you want to be in terms of fitness. Having a goal will also help keep your training routine a priority in your schedule. When you have an event to participate in, it helps you figure out how you can accomplish it.

Everyone is busy, but if you are working with other people towards an event, it can give you great motivation to train together. It builds camaraderie as you encourage each other to work harder or do better. Accomplishing a fitness goal for a charity, for example, may be challenging and rewarding at the same time. Here are some strategies to consider:

- Research an event or charity in your area
- Find out the particulars and sign up if you feel ready
- Mark the date on your calendar

- Share your goals with friends, family, and colleagues at work
- Calculate what you need to do to achieve your goal
- Schedule your workouts – treat them like an important meeting every week
- Are there others you can train with? It provides some healthy competition!

A week or so before your fitness event, wind back your training. This will allow you to begin at the starting line fresh and ready to take on the challenge. If you follow these strategies, the rest will take care of itself.

UNDERSTANDING THE GLYCEMIC INDEX

The Glycemic Index was first developed as a tool to help people control their blood sugar for diabetes. However, now it has come to the public arena and you can find low-glycemic cookbooks and meal plans everywhere. Some people swear by its value while others question if it is really necessary. The glycemic index measures how much a certain food will raise your blood sugar.

Foods with a higher GI value (greater than 70) tend to cause blood sugar levels to spike, including insulin, the hormone that helps glucose get into the cells. Blood sugar spikes are problematic for people dealing with diabetes and lack an effective insulin system to get rid of the sugar in the blood. Plus, higher GI foods tend to metabolized quickly, making you hungry again in an hour or sooner.

Lower GI foods are metabolized more slowly and can keep your appetite and blood sugar on a more even keel. Eating low glycemic index foods can help prevent damage to the cells caused by high blood-glucose concentrations. The controversy comes about because the glucose response to different foods varies widely from person to person. In other words, a low GI score is not guarantee of healthy fare. For example, a Coke can have a GI of 63 and potato chips are 54, so they might qualify as low or moderate GI — but they are not healthy choices.

The biggest problem is the GI looks at single foods; however, the real issue is what happens at mealtime. For example, if you add a pat of butter to a baked potato, that will slow down absorption of the potato's carbohydrate. While complex at times, this can be confusing to most people. In spite of these complications, following a low GI eating plan can help fine tune your meal plans and may even help you prevent diabetes in the future. Lower GI diets help lower the risk of:

- Age-related macular degeneration
- Heart disease

- Colorectal cancer
- Weight gain
- High cholesterol

The concept of following a meal plan with low GI foods makes sense. They are whole, natural, and unprocessed. Eating these types of foods is smart eating, no matter which side of the debate you are on.

THE TRUTH ABOUT GLUTEN

Many diseases have been linked to gluten. Gluten is a protein found in wheat, barley and rye. Many people with celiac disease or gluten intolerance are never diagnosed. Here are the signs and symptoms of gluten intolerance:

- Bloating
- Gas
- Diarrhea
- Constipation
- "Chicken Skin" on the back of the arms – known as keratosis pilaris and is a result of a vitamin A and fatty acid deficiency secondary to malabsorption of fat caused by gluten damaging the gut
- Brain fog
- Fatigue
- Feeling tired after eating a meal with gluten
- Diagnosis of an autoimmune disease including psoriasis, MS, rheumatoid arthritis, ulcerative colitis, Hashimoto's thyroiditis, and scleroderma
- Dizziness
- Hormone imbalances
- Unexplained infertility
- Migraine headaches
- Fibromyalgia
- Inflammation in the body
- Painful joints

- Anxiety
- Depression
- Mood swings
- ADD

The best way to determine if you are intolerant to gluten is to do an elimination diet. Remove gluten from your diet for at least two weeks, preferably three, and then reintroduce it. Gluten is a very large protein and it can take months and even years to clear it from your body. The longer you can take to eliminate it from your system, the better. If you notice that you feel better off gluten or feel worse when you introduce it, then gluten is probably an issue for you.

I am so tired of companies marketing gluten-free to people and acting like it is a healthy way of life if you don't have celiac disease. In reality gluten-free is not a diet. People think that if they are eating gluten-free that they will lose a ton of weight and are automatically being healthy. Just because brands advertise it on the front of their packaging with an underline or asterisk punctuation mark doesn't mean it's going to redefine your appearance.

IMPORTANCE OF LABELS AND SERVING SIZES

Learning to read labels makes it easier to use this information in the grocery store to make smart, quick, informed food choices that will contribute to your healthy diet. On the following page you will see a label for macaroni and cheese containing the serving size, calories, and nutrient information:

Nutrition Facts

Serving Size 2/3 cup (55g)
Servings Per Container About 8

Amount Per Serving

Calories 230   Calories from Fat 72

	% Daily Value*
Total Fat 8g	**12%**
Saturated Fat 1g	**5%**
Trans Fat 0g	
Cholesterol 0mg	**0%**
Sodium 160mg	**7%**
Total Carbohydrate 37g	**12%**
Dietary Fiber 4g	**16%**
Sugars 1g	
Protein 3g	

Vitamin A	10%
Vitamin C	8%
Calcium	20%
Iron	45%

* Percent Daily Values are based on a 2,000 calorie diet. Your daily value may be higher or lower depending on your calorie needs.

	Calories:	2,000	2,500
Total Fat	Less than	65g	80g
Sat Fat	Less than	20g	25g
Cholesterol	Less than	300mg	300mg
Sodium	Less than	2,400mg	2,400mg
Total Carbohydrate		300g	375g
Dietary Fiber		25g	30g

Begin With The Serving Size — This shows how many servings are in a package and, most importantly, how big the serving is. All the nutrition information on the label is based on that one serving of food. Of course, a package of food often contains more than one serving. If you eat **two servings** of the food, you are eating **double** the calories and getting **twice the amount** of nutrients, both good and bad.

Amount of Calories — The calories listed are for **one serving** of the food. "Calories from fat" shows how many fat calories there are in **one serving**. Remember: a product that's fat-free isn't necessarily calorie-free. Read the label.

Percent (%) Daily Value — This section tells you how the nutrients in one serving of the food contribute to your total daily diet. Use it to choose foods high in the nutrients you should get more of, and low in the nutrients you should minimize. Daily Values are based on a 2,000-calorie diet. However, your nutritional needs depend on how physically active you are.

Total Fat – You want to limit these nutrients, as eating too much total fat (especially saturated fat and trans fat), cholesterol, or sodium may increase your risk of certain chronic diseases, such as heart disease, some cancers, or high blood pressure. Try to keep these nutrients as low as possible each day.

Get Enough of These Nutrients

People often don't get enough dietary fiber, vitamin A, vitamin C, calcium, and potassium in their diets. These nutrients are essential for keeping you feeling strong and healthy. Eating enough of these nutrients may improve your health and help reduce the risk of some diseases.

Nutrients

A nutrient is an ingredient in a food that provides nourishment. Nutrients are essential for life and to keep your body functioning properly. There are some nutrients that are especially important for your health. You should try to get adequate amounts of these each day. They are:

- Calcium
- Dietary fiber
- Potassium
- Vitamin A
- Vitamin C

There are other important nutrients, you should eat in moderate amounts. They can increase your risk of certain diseases and include:

- Total fat (especially saturated fat)
- Cholesterol
- Sodium

The nutrition facts label can help you make choices for **overall health**. But some nutrients can also affect certain health **conditions and diseases**. Watch for "nutrients to get less of" (the ones that you should try to limit), and "nutrients to get more of" (the ones that are very important to be sure to get enough of) — the nutrition facts label is a tool that is available to you on every packaged food and beverage.

Vitamin Benefits and Program

First and foremost, a healthy diet is the foundation for good health, and taking a high-quality vitamin and mineral supplement will not make up for an unhealthy diet. That said, studies show that it's virtually impossible to get the breadth and levels of nutrients that you need for optimal health from diet alone. In fact, a USDA survey of almost 9,000 individuals showed that only a fraction of adults met adequate intake levels of essential nutrients like vitamin E, magnesium, vitamin A, and vitamin C. Additionally, nearly two-thirds of children fail to get Recommended Dietary Allowances (RDA) for vitamin E and zinc. Food Survey Research Groups have proven that half do not meet the RDA for calcium, and close to one-third fall short of the RDA for iron and vitamin B6. For these reasons, I'm a huge advocate of taking a pharmaceutical grade, clinically proven multivitamin like **Ferrigno FUEL** to fill in gaps and avoid the inevitable shortfalls from diet alone. I'm also a big fan of eating fresh fruits, vegetables, and whole grains as a baseline, as well as exercising and getting the proper amount of sleep.

Groups of people, from children to seniors and everyone in between, can benefit from taking our pharmaceutical-grade, clinically-proven supplements. So can those with eating disorders, people avoiding certain foods, vegetarians, and those with medical conditions or deficiency diseases. To reiterate, taking a good multivitamin means supplementing an already healthy diet and lifestyle to help fill in the gaps that you likely aren't getting through food alone. But not all supplements are created equal. While the FDA technically regulates the vitamin supplement industry, companies are allowed to self-police, which can lead to danger for consumers: from poor ingredient sourcing to fillers, additives, and more that can have a negative impact on the body.

How Can You Find A Great Multivitamin?

Advertising in the supplement industry can be incredibly creative and largely misleading. Avoid false promises by doing research on a particular vitamin or supplement brand. Make sure there is plenty of research supporting any claims, and ensure your supplement adheres to high-level manufacturing processes, is clinically proven, and only uses the best forms of ingredients. Here are some tips for selecting a supplement that is safe, effective, and, most importantly, will deliver on its health claims:

- Look for a supplement that is manufactured at pharmaceutical-grade standards.
- Is your supplement clinically proven? Not clinically tested, but clinically *proven*.
- Do the ingredients on the label match what's in the bottle?

- Does your supplement source the highest-quality, most bioavailable forms of each ingredient?

Why Pharmaceutical Grade?

I'm sorry if I am geeking out and mentioning the importance of pharmaceutical grade again, but I want to spend some time on why it is so important that your supplement adhere to those standards vs. Food Grade Standards. Pharmaceutical Grade manufacturing protocols ensure that supplements adhere to the same stringent production standards as the prescription drug industry. The majority of supplements on the market are sold at food grade standards, but by taking a pharmaceutical grade supplement you ensure your supplement is tested for dissolution and disintegration, and is required to dissolve within 45 minutes of ingesting the supplement. With food grade this is no dissolution requirement.

Pharmaceutical Grade standards also require that all raw materials are tested prior to production. This means testing for and removing any/all contaminants, bacteria, metals, microbials, etc. There is no raw materials testing requirement for food grade supplements, meaning contaminants may be present in your supplement. Finally, in pharmaceutical grade supplements it is required that the dosages and ingredients on the label match what is in the each and every capsule exactly. With food grade supplements the label is an approximation of what is in the capsules, and if your health matters to you I think you'd want to know exactly what you are putting into your body!

Always follow label directions and read the ingredient list and any warnings.

SUPPLEMENTS AND MEDICATION CAUTIONS

There are some dietary supplements that may interact with over-the-counter drugs or prescription medications. Take caution when taking supplements and medications at the same time. Here are some common interactions to watch out for:

- **Calcium** can interact with heart medicine, certain diuretics, and aluminum and magnesium-containing antacids.
- **Magnesium** can interact with certain diuretics, some cancer drugs, and magnesium-containing antacids.

- **Vitamin K** can interact with blood thinners like Coumadin.
- **St. John's Wort** is known to adversely affect selective serotonin reuptake inhibitor (SSRI) drugs (anti-depressant drugs), blood pressure medication, and birth control pills.
- **Coenzyme Q-10** can interact with anticoagulants, blood pressure medication, and chemotherapy drugs.
- **Ginkgo Biloba** and **Vitamin E** can increase the risk for internal bleeding when taken with aspirin or anticoagulants such as warfarin.
- **Ginseng** can also increase the risk for internal bleeding when taken with anticoagulants or NSAIDs, and may cause side effects when taken with MAOI antidepressants.
- **Echinacea** can change how the body breaks down certain medications in the liver.
- **Saw palmetto** can interact with anticoagulants and NSAID pain relievers.

MORE IS *NOT* ALWAYS BETTER

Even though our body can benefit from taking a certain supplement, in excessive doses, it is not a good idea. For example, taking high doses of green tea supplements can be highly toxic to the liver, as opposed to drinking green tea for its antioxidant and fat-burning benefits. Taking Vitamin E and selenium may increase the risk for prostate cancer in men. Ingesting high doses of Beta Carotene beyond the amount listed in your multi-vitamin and mineral can increase the risk for lung cancer in those that smoke.

Always follow label directions and read the ingredient list and any warnings.

CLIENT STORY: AARON

Age: 24
Height: 5′4″
Weight before: 252 lbs

How I gained weight: As long as I can remember I have been overweight. When I was a child, I remember having to buy "Husky-sized" clothes, but never really thought anything of it. Kids can't be overweight, right? I played sports like baseball, football, and soccer so there really wasn't a point before high school where I felt that my weight was ever a concern. My mom cooked home meals often and that is what I understood what made a healthy person. As long as you're not eating fast food on a regular basis you're eating healthy. Lasagna, pizza, and burgers were my personal favorites. Nothing would beat my mom's homemade BBQ chicken with mashed potatoes.

Obviously, now I have a better understanding that destroys that logic but it's not like school talks to a bunch of preteens about calories and how food and exercise affects your body. At least, in the early 1990s they didn't. Sure, there was P.E. class, but all we ever did was play games and jump rope.

As a kid, I idolized my dad. He was popular in school, an amazing athlete and a great person. That's when I started playing football, so I could be more like him and let him live through me vicariously. But it was short lived and I went back to just playing percussion in middle school band and didn't focus on sports much.

My opinion on my appearance really didn't affect me until I was a freshman in high school. I look edaround me and there were all these fit teenagers and I was the overweight band nerd. Around the same time, I went on the Atkins diet. I ate all the meat and cheese I wanted to lose weight; seemed pretty ideal to me. But when that eventually failed, I moved on from trying to lose weight and just loved myself for who I was.

That's what I heard all the time. "Don't hate yourself. Embrace how you look and don't change for anyone." I was bullied a lot in school. Random upperclassmen I didn't even know would ridicule me, call me names. There was even a time in school I was walking down the hall during class and this random senior slapped me in the face, laughed, and walked on. I stayed the course of my terrible eating habits and graduated high school weighing over 200 pounds at 5'4".

After high school, I slowly but surely started to gain some serious weight. Every day I was eating Taco Bell and McDonald's while playing video games online — literally wasting away in front of a TV. Once I noticed my weight going up I started dieting again. I would drop about 20 pounds, hit a wall, and then go back to my normal eating habits. I went through this cycle at least 4 times that I can remember. Not being able to keep the weight off just added to the depression I was battling at the time so food was a pretty good answer for combating those troubles.

It got to the point that I was lying to myself, saying, "I have maintained the same weight since high school. No need for me to lose any weight. I'm the same size at 20 that I was when I was 17." I knew that was a lie, but it made me feel better about my weight. You know when they say if you keep telling yourself a lie over and over, eventually you believe it? That was where I was with my weight. "Well, if I were taller, it wouldn't seem so bad."

I had very little guidance when it came to getting motivated and losing weight. I remember one time I was at the gym, a regular gym rat saw me doing leg presses and just started laughing at me. Who wouldn't be discouraged at that? I thought that he would have motivated me because I was trying to better myself. I didn't see the point of trying anymore. Why diet when I knew I was going to fail? Why go to the gym if even there you get laughed at? So I just went back to eating what I want and kept telling myself that I was happy.

Breaking point: Then there I was. 24 years old and over 250 pounds. "What the hell happened?" I asked myself. I would remember when I could fit my XL shirts just fine; all of a sudden, they were too tight and too revealing. So I had to go up to XXL. I realized how I would lose my breath just going up the stairs or even getting into bed. I would look down and barely be able to see my feet. I cried. I cried for so long and so hard. My dad told me when I was young, "Don't cry unless you are in serious pain or if you have lost someone close to you." Now, he said that with all the love you would want and need from a father — and I remember thinking that I am in pain and I have lost someone.

I was in physical and emotional pain from where I was at in my weight, and I had lost the person I used to be. I started to wonder, if I go to sleep, would I wake up? You hear about overweight people dying in their sleep all the time. For me, it was a real possibility and it terrified me. I was tired of feeling unattractive, knowing that people talked about me behind my back. I saw my dad lose a ton of weight and I knew that if he could do it, I could too. No more backing down or making excuses. I wanted this damn weight off of me.

How I lost the weight: It first started out by simply counting calories and monitoring what I ate. With my new job, I was literally walking upwards of 6 miles a day so I knew that I could just start focusing on my eating habits. But, then I started getting back to my old ways. With no guidance on proper eating behavior or how to make food work for you, it's hard to just simply watch what you eat. Then, I looked up Ferrigno FIT online. I remembered seeing the logo on an episode of Comic Book Men when Lou Ferrigno made an appearance.

After doing some research on what was provided, I took a leap and signed up. After that, my life was changed. I had a meal plan to follow so I wasn't blindly trying to put together meals and it was the right food for losing weight. I started the home workout films that were provided. The first time through, I would take frequent water breaks. But, I at least pushed myself to get through the workout.

By the end of the first week, I was able to get through without stopping. I completed the 12-week program, getting thinner and stronger every day. Now, I go to the gym regularly and eat without a meal plan because I have the knowledge needed to make conscious decisions on my meals. I still walk, on average 7-8 miles a day, and run at the gym. The whole time I had the support of my amazing fiancé, my family, and my friends.

After weight: I am currently 175 pounds with 15 pounds of it as added muscle weight. I went from a XXL to a Medium. I will never forget that moment. I stood in the dressing room and the department store and just cried. As much as I tried not to, I just couldn't hold it in. My pants went from a 44-inch waist to 32-inch waist. Every day, I push myself 110% for my family and myself. I am going back to school for Nutritional Science and Personal Training so I can help other people just like me. After all, I needed to be inspired to stay motivated. So why not pass it along?

EXCUSE #6:
I HAVE TOO MANY RESPONSIBILITIES

We are all busy, with many responsibilities and worthy needs to address every day. Many people, especially women, have trouble prioritizing their health in their day-to-day routine. This chapter discusses why taking care of yourself ultimately allows you to take better care of others, if you are choosing to do that, and helps the reader strategize on how to deal with any disruptions their new routines may be causing among friends and family members. It also discusses the relationship of sleep to both exercise performance and weight loss.

You are stepping up your workouts this week! Reflect on how you felt while you were increasing your steps last week and when you did the cardio piece of your fitness assessment. If you are a beginner, challenge yourself to WALK ONE MILE, BRISKLY, 3-5 TIMES THIS WEEK. That should ideally take you no more than 15 or 20 minutes, so it's not going to be a huge time suck. If it's taking you longer, don't worry, just walk as fast as you can and see if you can drop your time this week, even by a little bit.

If you are more intermediate, but new to running, I want you to RUN FOR 2 MINUTES AND THEN WALK FOR TWO MINUTES, REPEATING THAT PATTERN FOR AT LEAST ONE MILE OR HALF AN HOUR, whichever feels reasonably challenging. If you want to do this three times this week and walk briskly on two other days, that's also a fine goal. The point is to keep yourself challenged. You need a stopwatch or a stopwatch function on your smartphone to do this.

EXAMINING WHAT YOU TOLERATE

We are all creatures of habit. In fact, for better or worse, some of our habits are on automatic pilot. Your successes with *The Reset Plan* will be directly related to your habits and are the product of your beliefs. In order to enjoy some healthy permanent changes in your life, you must change any negative beliefs and the habits that go with them. From the moment you wake up in the morning, your habits are in place, often with little thought or consideration. The state of your body and health reflects your exercise and eating habits. These habits either serve you or they do not. They can take you away from your intended outcome or bring you closer. Recognizing and knowing your beliefs about your habits is the key to changing your bad ones.

Your actions and thoughts reflect your beliefs. You cannot expect to make permanent changes in your health and body if your underlying belief about change is negative. In order to transform any bad habits and change them into positive ones, you must also change your beliefs. Changing habits and changing beliefs go hand in hand.

Trying to establish new habits without dealing with any underlying negative belief makes it difficult to change any negative habits. Underlying negative beliefs are the source of your failed attempts to make positive changes. For example, the main reason why most diets fail is because the dieter has a negative underlying belief that goes unchecked. If the dieter believes he or she is fat, for example, then no exercise or good health program will create any permanent success if that belief remains the same. Sooner or later, actions will be taken to fulfill the negative belief. Keep in mind — slim people do not "diet."

If you are trying to create a positive new habit while still holding on to a negative belief, that takes a tremendous amount of willpower and your success is not likely. However, once you change the negative belief that goes along with your negative habit, changing habits is much easier. In other words, creating a new healthy habit requires little or no willpower when your underlying belief is working with it instead of against it.

You don't have to wait any longer to change your beliefs before creating healthy new habits. Changing any negative beliefs you may have first before changing any habits is important. Change the two together and you will be successful. Changing your belief from "I am overweight" to "I am slim and healthy," while at the same time adopting healthy exercise and eating habits that reflect this new belief, is the best way to achieve permanent success.

Over the years, both your good and bad habits were created from the beliefs you adopted through interactions with your parents, family, friends, peers, teachers, and society in general. Social conditioning has a profound effect on your beliefs and habits. Consciously, look at the habits that serve you and eliminate those habits that fail you by changing your beliefs. It is never too late to change your health, exercise and eating habits. All of your habits live in your subconscious mind where you no longer think about them. Changing habits permanently involves reprogramming your unwanted negative beliefs at the subconscious level.

One of the best ways to change habits successfully is through creative visualization. You can change any negative belief by visualizing yourself experiencing the new positive belief repeatedly. Soon, you will find that your thoughts and actions in your day-to-day life begin to reflect those new beliefs until they become a healthy new habit. Be aware that visualizing an intended outcome without dealing with any negative beliefs can derail your efforts and attract more of what you don't want.

When changing your negative habits, you will know how much your underlying negative beliefs have been replaced by gauging how much willpower you have to use. Any time you have to use significant amounts of willpower to do something healthy or positive you know will serve you, there may be a major conflict between your underlying negative beliefs and your actions. In other words, anything you say or do that is aligned with your beliefs should not require much effort. Your aim is to transform your actions into healthy habits of your subconscious mind that does not require willpower.

If you can repeat a healthy habit often enough without having to consciously think about it is a testament to the power of your mind. This new ability can make it easier to learn new information that serves your success until your actions become habitual and the process can be repeated again and again. You can choose beliefs and habits that will serve you and your success. You have the power to create a healthy life.

To quote Gandhi,

"Your **beliefs** become your **thoughts.**

Your thoughts become your **words.**

Your words become your **actions.**

Your actions become your **habits.**

Your habits become your **values.**

Your values become your **destiny.**"

The state of your health is really a reflection of the actions, words, and thoughts you repeat subconsciously. Let's face it: we are all creatures of habit. However, your life is a reflection of those habits, which are in turn a product of your beliefs. Most people make the effort to change any negative habits without considering or facing the underlying negative belief. However, by reprogramming your beliefs, you can create new healthy habits that will contribute to your successful eating and exercising and eliminate habits that do not.

LEARNING HOW TO SAY *NO* WITHOUT ANGER OR GUILT

Saying "no" to unhealthy urges can be quite freeing. It allows you to use your mind to make a smart decision rather than being at the mercy of every whim or craving. The word "discipline" comes from the word "disciple" which means "learner." You must be willing to learn. Most people do not like idea of feeling controlled or restrained and generally look at freedom in a positive light. What you may not realize is that discipline can ultimately lead to freedom, and can help you achieve your heart's desire.

Taking care of your body and treating it with respect can allow the physical and spiritual worlds to meet. Taking care of your mind, body, and spirit will help you function at optimum levels all around and be of service to others. Ancient traditions such as yoga and Tai Chi are based on self-disciplines emphasizing a daily practice that perfects the art. However, any activity requiring focus on the mind and body such as swimming, weight training, gardening, or even surfing can support self-mastery of that endeavor. Engage in activities that make you feel good about "you."

MAKING TIME FOR YOURSELF IS NECESSARY, NOT SELFISH

Have you ever wished you had more time to yourself? Do you often say you wish there are more hours in a day or you don't have time for an activity? We all lead busy lives, but the one thing we do not take time for are ourselves. It seems like we are always juggling family, work, spouse, social life, and other demands on our time. However, when we take the time to pursue our passion, do what we enjoy doing, or even relax and do nothing at all, we feel better.

Taking time for yourself allows you to unwind, rejuvenate, and de-stress. Taking time for yourself allows you to heal and be peaceful. Most people feel like it is selfish to take "me"-time, or feel guilty for doing so. The more caring and giving a person you are, the more these guilty feelings seem to emerge. Even though there are only 24 hours in a day, you can clear some time for yourself by reevaluating your priorities. Practice some smart time management or simply say "no."

Do not feel guilty for "me"-time; when our schedules become out of balance, our energy drops. Lowered energy creates the illusion there isn't enough time in the day, so a vicious cycle of time limitation continues. Adding regular doses of "me"-time to your day and will allow you to come back to your responsibilities with greater commitment, enjoyment, and focus. It is quite common, especially for women, to be so involved in giving to others and our families we fail to give to ourselves. Men can feel this way, too — getting so caught up in making a living that they rarely take time to hang out with the guys, pursue a hobby, or simply read. Make time for yourself, and do not feel guilty about it.

IMPORTANCE OF STARTING INSIDE OUT

Many of my clients who have seen a transformation in their bodies realize the changes took place from the inside out. What they observe on the outside is really a reflection of the changes that occurred on the inside. While many are concerned about losing body fat too slowly, all of my clients feel better and have more energy simply by weight training and doing cardiovascular exercises, in spite of feeling a bit sore.

You must understand that fat is stored in several places including within the muscle, around the organs (known as "visceral fat") and under the skin (known as subcutaneous fat). Weight training tends to draw from the intramuscular stores early on, and instead of seeing a major change in the mirror, you might feel your muscles getting firm. This is a good sign. Do not give up. The subcutaneous fat loss becomes more noticeable once the intramuscular stores are whittled down.

Many of my women clients who have large thighs, hips, and calves are concerned weight training will make them larger. Nothing could be further from the truth. The muscles in your thighs, hips, and calves are most likely marbleized with fat. Weight training allows the muscles to become more elongated rather than bulky. Lifting weights allows you to lose body fat and support and maintain muscle. You must understand that by lifting weights, your muscles store more glycogen. Every gram of glycogen binds to water within the muscle, and that is what bodybuilders refer to as "getting a pump." Regular exercise increases blood volume, and so initially your weight loss efforts may not show up on the scale. Believe me, there are days you will wake up and notice big changes, and other days where it seems like nothing is happening.

Hang in there and stay with it. Results will come.

For many people, the initial drop that shows on the scale will understate your fat loss in the first few weeks. In fact, if you have a lot of weight to lose, the drop on the scale will most likely exceed your fat loss. This is quite common if your diet was high in carbohydrates before you started *The Reset Plan*. Many people think water loss is not true weight loss. If your body fat level stays the same, that is true. However, water retention is determined by the amount of your body fat; if you lose the fat, the water stays off as well.

Do not ignore increases and improvements in strength and overall feeling of wellbeing. If you could look inside your body, you would see, as a result of your changes made:

- "Good" enzymes increasing in the cells

136

- Energy-producing mitochondria multiplying
- Lowered cholesterol
- Arteries becoming more clear
- Blood vessels working more efficiently
- Stronger muscles
- Improved bone density

The Reset Plan will create all these incredible and significant internal changes as progress on the outside continues to accelerate. Some people experience more internal changes than others, due to years of yo-yo dieting, prior lifestyle habits and other considerations. Know that if you are following the program, the progress is happening, whether it is obvious to you or not. Follow your *Reset Plan* consistently. Review your workouts. Troubleshoot. You will succeed.

THE SCIENCE OF SLEEP

Most workout programs do not focus on sleep. No doubt you will notice you are sleeping well soon after starting *The Reset Plan*. What you need to be aware of is not to push yourself too hard and not get enough sleep. Getting enough sleep actually helps your fitness program and health. When you get enough sleep, you will feel more rested and ready to give it your all during your workout. It is impossible to make improvements in your physique and fitness level without enough sleep.

Sleep helps the body's chemical processes work better. For example, your muscles are allowed to repair and build up during sleep which is why it is important to get enough protein during the day. In fact, what you eat and drink during the day can affect the quality of your sleep tremendously. When you don't get enough sleep, it is the same as overtraining your body.

Your body, including your brain, is worn out, rather than built up, if you are lacking sleep. The endorphin "high" that comes with fitness workouts comes more easily after a good night's sleep. If you are not sleeping well night after night, it can put you in a bad mood and makes it difficult to stay motivated and focused with *The Reset Plan*. It is always easier to stay on your eating plan if you are well-rested.

When you are extremely tired, you tend to rely on comfort foods and that usually means too many carbohydrates, not enough lean protein, and too much fat. Aim for at least 7-9 hours of sleep every night. A good night's sleep will go a long way in helping you stay with *The Reset Plan* and less likely to cheat. Sleep is often the missing ingredient in health and fitness programs.

FIGURING OUT WHAT MAKES YOU LOOK (AND FEEL) GOOD

The rewards of being consistent with *The Reset Plan* go far beyond adding muscle tone and losing weight. You will notice several subtle changes that affect both your mind and body. You might notice you are sleeping better when it used to be elusive for you. Your skin looks better and your eyes are brighter. These little victories are just as valid as the gains measured by the scale or skin calipers.

Every cell in your body benefits from regular exercise — within one hour of finishing your workout, you feel less stressed, calm, can sleep better, and your body will process blood sugar more efficiently. Here are just a few ways that *The Reset Plan* can make you look and feel good:

More Radiant Skin — Working up a good sweat is like getting a mini-facial. Your pores dilate, and the sweat expels trapped oil and dirt. Of course, it is always a good idea to wash your face after a hard workout.

Reduces Inflammation — Throughout the body, helping to regulate significant hormones in the skin and prevents free-radical damage. Exercise revs up your skin's collagen production, and in the process helps to prevent wrinkles and makes your skin look younger.

Feel Better About Your Self-Worth — This is directly tied to our energy levels and perceived attractiveness. We feel more confident and competent after exercise. There is nothing more attractive than feel self-assured in your own skin.

Stand Taller — Exercise actually stretches and strengthens your muscles at the same time. Adding yoga and Pilates to your workout can improve posture and therefore add height. When you actively bring your muscles back into balance, your back will lengthen and your posture will improve. Plus, it tends to make you look fitter, taller, and more confident.

Feeling Less Stressed — Stress can definitely show up on your face and regular exercise can alleviate most mild to moderate stress levels and improve your mood. The calming effect can last for hours.

Builds Your Immune System — Exercise enhances your immune system by prompting the body to churn out more white blood cells, including natural killer cells. More white blood cells mean fewer viruses and bacteria sneak past the gate, so to speak. Wounds heal faster and the lymph system is happier. When muscles contract during exercise, they put the squeeze on lymph nodes, helping them to pump waste out of your system.

Better Sleep — Exercise sharpens the body's sensitivity to the stress hormone cortisol that can enhance sleep. When you are stressed out and if it is chronic, and you do not exercise, the cortisol stays in the blood. Exercise is basically a release valve for cortisol, allowing you to sleep better and more soundly, leaving you looking healthy and fresh.

Lose Those Love Handles — Losing excess body fat deep inside the body boosts your overall vitality and looks. Regular exercise trains the body to burn visceral fat more efficiently.

Look And Feel More Sexy — Exercise balances the body's sex hormones, which in turn can improve the appearance of your skin, muscle tone and hair.

All of these benefits add up to making you feel and look good. Exercise is not just about burning more calories. It is so much more once you factor in reduced stress, better sleep, and enjoying an overall healthy body.

LOOKING YOUNGER WITH NATURAL FOODS

Fresh fruits, vegetables, and nuts contain powerful anti-aging chemicals that make you look and feel younger. For example, nuts contain essential fatty acids responsible for maintaining healthy cells. They can help prevent toxins from entering the cells. Lemons and other citrus fruits cleanse and nourish the skin. Avocado is rich in healthy natural oils and good fats that are excellent for the skin. Spend some time in the produce section and build a meal around fresh fruits and vegetables. Eating natural, whole foods promotes general well-being, weight loss, and helps give your skin a natural glow. Here are some more tips and suggestions for looking younger with natural organic foods:

Limit Your Salt Intake — If you must add salt to your food or while cooking, make sure you use Himalayan Pink Salt, which is full of natural minerals that will not elevate blood pressure. Iodized salt causes water retention and elevates blood pressure. Cutting down on salt can make you feel less heavy and sluggish. Ready-to-eat meals, breads and soups contain a lot of salt.

Get Your Antioxidants — These are found in fresh fruits and vegetables and serve up plenty of health benefits including the prevention of many cancers.

Choose Organic — This will reduce your exposure to pesticides found on commercial produce. Pesticides are becoming a factor contributing to ADHD, autism, and other neurological impairments in children.

Avoid Exposure To Antibiotics — The increasing use of antibiotics among feedlots and dairy farms is a huge concern for all of us in the U.S. Organically raised animals are not given antibiotic additives. Consistent exposure to antibiotic residue can disrupt the normal flora of the human gut, reducing the amount of healthy bacteria and leaving us more vulnerable to harmful illness and bacteria.

Know About GMOs — There has been an increase in production of genetically modified foods and the lack of labeling of these foods is cause for concern. GMO foods can depress the immune system and cause reproductive dysfunction, allergies, cancer, and high toxicity levels in the body. Over 70% of all processed foods contain GM ingredients, even if it is organic. Stay away from processed foods.

THE COSMETIC INDUSTRY

It is always a good idea to put more thought into your appearance, especially as you continue to improve your physique and health. Let's face it: the fashion and cosmetic industry have become billion-dollar industries. People have a hard time looking past a sloppy exterior. Why not live up to and maximize your appearance's full potential and get your act together on the outside? When you look like you have your act together, others can't help but believe you do. However, the opposite is true if you dress sloppily, don't wear any make-up, or don't fix your hair.

It is time to clean up your look, which will enhance how you feel from the inside out. Good grooming will go a long way in not selling yourself short. Improving your appearance can have a dramatic effect on your social life. Outward appearances really do play a strong role in social situations.

There are no downsides to improving your look. You can also have fun in becoming more fashionable than you have been in the past. Yes — you will have to learn about style and clothes, devote some of your time to shopping and probably spend some money. Looking half-decent does not mean you need to change everything about your appearance. Your current style may be just fine, or you may want to get an outside opinion from a stylist or fashion expert.

Once you devote a little time and thought as to how you look, you can easily correct any of the following:

Groom Your Hair — This goes for guys, too, and even includes taming your eyebrows. Washing your hair regularly is a given — you have to do it.

Use A Good Moisturizer On Your Skin — There are many on the market today and sampling different ones or getting a facial with recommendations for skincare is important.

Brush And Floss Your Teeth Daily — Most dentists recommend brushing after every meal or at least twice a day.

Be Conscious Of Your Breath — Brush your tongue and use breath mints if necessary.

Shower Or Take A Bath Daily — Taking a bath at night before bed is a great way to calm your body and cleanse yourself from the day.

Trim Your Toenails and Fingernails — Schedule a manicure or pedicure (or both) on a consistent basis.

Find The Best-Looking Hairstyle For Your Face — This might mean getting a haircut or growing your hair out. Good-looking hair is really the cornerstone of an attractive appearance and can have the most impact when you make a first impression on someone.

ARE YOU ADDICTED TO COUNTING CALORIES?

I hear a lot of chatter from my clients about counting calories, like "I can have this because it is only 200 calories" or "I was on the treadmill today for 40 minutes so I can eat 600 calories at dinner." It is almost like my clients look at calories like money where they exchange food choices and exercises for calories consumed. In other words, they often judge their success and failure based on whether or not they reached or met their caloric limit for the day.

We can get down on ourselves if we couldn't resist dessert or didn't exercise long enough. Many of my clients visualize calories going straight to their hips if they don't keep tabs on them. It can leave them feeling disempowered, deflated and defeated. Counting calories was something I did myself in my early years. In fact, I was so preoccupied with hitting the right number of calories for my height and weight, I stopped listening to my body.

Relying on an iPad, phone, or calorie counter to tell me what to eat left me feeling deprived and starved. I lost touch with my taste buds and hunger cues and would reach for any product that was labeled "low-calorie" or "low-fat." My meals were full of artificial foods instead of "real" foods. Plus, calorie counting is exhausting. All of this obsessive behavior was not doing anything for my vitality and health. My hair was thinning, I had no energy, and I could not lose weight. Does any of this sound familiar?

It is time to get back in tune with your body and learn to eat when you are hungry. Trust your body and learn to enjoy foods without experiencing guilt. Real food — food your grandmother would be proud to serve on her dinner table — is the key to good health. Learn to thrive from food produced by Mother Earth. Here are some tips to make a change that will help you:

Eat From The Earth — Focus on ingredients instead of the calories. Know where your food comes from. Support local farmers markets and fill up on foods that are nutrient-dense.

Choose Foods You CAN Pronounce — If a food has more than 5 ingredients and an expiration date far in the future, you do not want to eat it, especially if you cannot pronounce an ingredient.

Enjoy Healthy Fats — Like those from olive oil, avocados and nuts. Coconut oil and the natural fats from healthy organic dairy products and animals will support the health of your body.

Make Note Of How A Food Makes You Feel — Reflect back on how you feel after eating a meal. Are you energized or want to lie down and take a nap?

Learn To Eat Slowly — Savor your food instead of eating something in your car driving down the freeway.

Explore Your Relationship With Food — Be honest with yourself. If you are not getting the results despite your efforts, we may need to fine-tune your eating plan.

Do not be afraid to reach out to me for help. It is a process and totally worth it. You will find freedom when you look at food for nourishment rather than asking if it is low in calories. It might mean identifying a food that triggers a craving, for example. Whatever it is, we can figure it out. You are not alone.

THE SCALE – WHY WE ARE ADDICTED TO THE NUMBERS GAME

The thought of weighing yourself may seem like a daunting task, which is why I encouraged you earlier on to put it away or ditch it all together. If you still have the need to hold onto your scale and don't believe you have a problem with it, make sure you think about the scale as a compass to make sure you are headed in the right direction. It can tell us if we need to modify your eating plan or exercises to ensure successful results.

Here are some tips to consider if you must weigh yourself:

Do NOT Weigh Yourself Every Day — Your weight fluctuates throughout the day due to fluid fluctuations in the body. Minor fluctuations can freak you out or base your whole day on what the scale says. Instead, judge yourself on how your clothes are fitting and endurance levels.

Weigh Yourself Once A Week — Choose a day that works well for you and will give you an accurate reading. It is realistic to lose ½ to 1 pound per week and will help you figure out if you need to make adjustments with your program.

Face The Scale — But only once a week. Not weighing yourself at all is not a good idea either. It is important to know what the number is on the scale and if you need to make some changes. It is a good way to keep tabs on yourself and your progress. With that said, as you lift weights and support more lean muscle tissue, the effects may not always show on the scale. In other words, you will look slimmer or smaller in your arms, hips and abs, for example, but this may not be reflected in the number on the scale. Do not be discouraged; women tend to hold on to water to heal during the weight training process. Eventually, the bloat will dissipate and you are left with a lean, toned body.

FOCUS: Make sure you are using the scale for the right reason.

INVEST: Take note of how you are feeling when you do weigh yourself.

TAKE ACTION: Remember, the scale is a machine with an opinion. Just like everyone will have an opinion about you, you have to be clear about yourself to take it all with a grain of salt.

CELEBRITY STORY: NICOLE SCHERZINGER

When clients come to me and say they want to look like a certain celebrity, I always tell them to focus on loving their own mind and body. In other words, you never know what that celebrity might be battling to look a certain way. Take, for example, Nicole Scherzinger, the former Pussycat Doll singer. She is known for her amazing voice, powerful presence, and incredible dance moves, giving the impression that she has it all.

However, the X-Factor judge has shared her experiences of struggling with bulimia that began in her twenties. She knew, in order to live a happy, healthy life, that she would need professional help to overcome this debilitating condition. Feeling miserable on the inside with a great life on the outside just doesn't work. Her family hid it well but she knew this eating disorder was not normal and had to do something about it.

Losing her voice, not being able to sing or handle the long, grueling hours of rehearsal and show tours, she knew that if she didn't get help, she would lose everything she had worked so hard to attain. She had to find a way to love herself. As a result of speaking out about her eating disorder, she has helped many dealing with a similar situation find a solution. You, too, can recover from an eating disorder and learn to love yourself. Her message of love and empathy has gone a long way in helping people beat bulimia once and for all. Do not be ashamed — you are loved.

EXCUSE #7:
NO ONE UNDERSTANDS ME

Think about the last time you were misunderstood. What were the feelings that came up the most and how did you handle it? 80% of clients who walk through my door identify with the feeling of being misunderstood. Unless you have a kick-ass support system in your life, this feeling can be turned on you as an excuse to why you are not "taking care of yourself."

There are two HUGE beliefs I have in life, no matter the scenario:

1. If you haven't walked in a person's shoes you should not feel like you have any right to judge them.

2. You can NEVER debate a person's feelings. How a person feels is their right to have, whether you feel they are making an excuse or not. They are entitled to their feelings.

When people make big changes in their lives, most are being genuinely misunderstood — and not supported — by important people in their lives. This chapter addresses both scenarios, with an action plan and responses that will help make your efforts to get healthy successful.

We have to stop believing from society that things will magically be different in our lives if we could just lose the weight. A lot of gates do open on the physical side, in a positive way, when people lose a great deal of weight — but you don't become a different person. You're still you — and you still have the same insecurities as before — which is why it's so important to *Reset* from the inside out.

HAVING THE RIGHT DIALOGUE WITH YOURSELF

Long-term, successful weight loss starts in your head. Having the right attitude can help you "think yourself lean." If you want to be successful with your weight loss, you need to look at the habits and patterns in your life getting in the way of your success. When trying to improve diet and lifestyle, most people do okay until some life event occurs that they can't control, and triggers them back to their old patterns.

Weight loss is usually slow and many people do not have the patience to stick with it; they want instant gratification and immediate results. But you did not put weight on overnight, so do not expect to lose weight overnight. However, you will get the best weight loss results when you lose it slowly. If you lose weight fast, you are usually losing lean muscle tissue and water, not body fat. When you lose lean muscle tissue, your metabolism slows down, making it even harder to lose weight.

Here are some tips and suggestions to think about that will enhance your weight loss efforts:

Visualize Yourself LEAN — Think about how good you will look with those extra pounds gone. Look for old photographs of yourself when you were slimmer as a reminder of what you are working towards. In order to break old habits, you need to see yourself in a positive light. Think back to when you were at your happiest weight. How old were you? Where were you in life mentally and physically?

Be Realistic — If you want to lose 20 pounds and you can look ahead in one year, then that is really only 1-2 pounds per month — something doable and manageable, even with a busy lifestyle. Like they say in AA: one day at a time. I believe the same is true with food addictions. If you don't go moment-by-moment you are going to give up when you're having a bad day and daunted by doughnuts. Stay in the moment and slay one goal at a time.

Set Mini-Goals — Make a list of mini-goals to help you reach your weight loss goals. Do little things, such as eating more fruits and vegetables or getting more physical activity in your day. Order a side salad instead of french fries. Take the stairs instead of the elevator at work. Change is hard, but it can be even more difficult if we try and make too many changes at once. Start small and gradually make lifestyle improvements.

Connect With Others — Instead of trying to go it alone, find someone you can connect with on your weight loss journey. Of course, I am always here for you.

Make Your Health a Priority in Your Life — Every night, plan your healthy meals and schedule your workouts as if you are making an appointment with yourself. Pack up some healthy snacks to take with you to work. Ultimately, these healthy behaviors will become a routine in your life.

Reward Yourself for Achieving a Mini-Goal — Get a manicure, pedicure, facial, or get your hair done. Celebrate the little steps you achieve in your weight loss efforts. Just like a recovering alcoholic wouldn't celebrate a 30-day chip with a glass of wine, don't reward yourself with food.

Identify Your Behaviors That Lead To Weight Gain — For example, if you are used to watching TV with a bag of potato chips, enjoy an apple with almond butter instead. If you're really craving chips and an apple and almond butter just won't do it alone one day, grab a handful of potato chips and put them on a plate. Ditch eating out of the bag; portion your serving and enjoy each chip at a time. At this point, you should know how hard you are physically working to burn it off, so enjoy every crunch. Do leg lifts or squats while watching television. Get rid of the empty-calorie foods in your house and replace them with healthier options.

Keep A Journal — Knowing that you are tracking your food intake can help you resist dessert, especially when you know you have to write it down. Keeping a journal helps you understand *you* — your emotions, how much exercise you are getting, and details what you are eating. A journal will help you figure out which strategies are working and which are not.

REDEFINING FAILURE AND FEAR

You might be thinking, "How hard can it be to eat right, exercise and get enough sleep to lose weight?" However, many people gain weight because they:

- Overestimate how much they exercise versus calories burned
- Skip meals
- Underestimate how many calories are being consumed
- Do not get enough sleep

Selecting foods that will keep you full instead of those lacking nutrients and leave you feeling hungry is a great goal to focus on. You should not deprive yourself and you need to eat when you are hungry. Incorporate a variety of foods that include protein, fats and carbohydrates. A good day of meals would include a Western omelet with a ½ cup of berries for breakfast; a ground turkey patty with a baked sweet potato topped with cinnamon and grilled vegetables for lunch;

dinner might be grilled shrimp or fish with steamed broccoli served over a bed of spaghetti squash tossed with olive oil, garlic and herbs. The point is to not fear food. It nourishes your body and can help you lose weight when you eat right.

If you get hungry between meals, have a cup of plain Greek yogurt or cottage cheese with some berries, an apple with almond butter, or celery sticks dipped in peanut butter. For successful weight loss, your diet counts more than exercise. However, be active and enjoy your exercise.

Get in the habit of listening to your body. Focus on increasing your awareness of your own hunger, which is your body's way of telling you when it needs food. When you are hungry, do not look at it as being a failure — instead use it as a chance to fuel your body with healthy choices.

When it comes to sleep, turn your bedroom into a sleeping sanctuary, making it as comfortable and dark as possible for a good night's sleep. Turn the computer off at 9:00 p.m. and avoid caffeine, supplements, lots of beverages, or medicines at least two hours before you plan to go to bed. You have nothing to lose but weight.

Identifying Who The Enablers Are In Your Life

You have been working hard to lose weight and striving to make real changes in how you eat, exercise, and live so you can be happy and healthy while maintaining your weight loss. You have friends and family who are supporting you and are on your side, but you are beginning to wonder who is really on your side. However, have you noticed some people in your life are resistant to the positive changes you are making in your life? Are some people encouraging you to slide back into old unhealthy behaviors? They may not mean to do it, but some people you love may be enabling bad behaviors. In order to change, you need to address this issue.

What Is An Enabler?

An enabler is someone who allows you to get away with eating unhealthy by taking away any of the consequences. This person may love you and think they are helping you. Enablers can influence all kinds of negative behaviors. You might have a friend you like to go shopping with and she always wants to have dessert instead of just a cup of coffee. It is up to you to recognize any enablers in your life.

They are not bad people, but their actions may keep you from making the positive changes you need to lose weight and keep it off. He or she may makes excuses for you when you fail to reach your weight loss goal, or, when you set specific goals for a healthy meal, the enabler tells you you don't need to eat that.

It can be tough to spot an enabler because they seem like they are all about love. However, when you need to lose weight and make changes in your life, you need some tough love. You need those in your life who are honest with you and tell you when you mess up, so you can experience the consequences of your bad food choices.

How to *RESET* An Enabler

Once you realize who might be an enabler in your life, it is time to sit down and have a talk. Remember: this person loves you, but probably does not realize how they might be sabotaging your weight loss efforts. Explain to this person they are making it more difficult for you to lose weight when they keep suggesting a dessert or talking about food all the time. Share specific examples and explain how you need to change. Be sensitive but firm.

If you find after several attempts to discuss this with the enabler and nothing changes, you may need to distance yourself from that person for a period of time. You can't let the enabler hold you back from making positive, healthy changes, especially when your health is on the line. A little distance from this person may be all you need and can make all the difference.

Identifying Who Emotional Vampires Are

Do you ever feel physically or emotionally drained after spending time with someone? Does your anxiety level go up? Do you feel sad or depressed for no reason? These are all red flags that are signaling you to run from these emotional vampires that can suck the very life out of you. Recognizing these difficult people is the first step in preparing yourself to handle them properly and effectively to diffuse them or the situation.

Losing weight is tough enough without dragging yourself through dirt and grime created by emotional vampires hidden where you least expect them. There is only one way to handle emotional vampires: remove the difficult person from your presence and make room for the positive you will gain. The choice is yours to make. If you prefer sunny skies over cloudy days and dealing with smiles instead of difficult personalities, emotional vampires in your life need your undivided attention. Take action now and you will win at weight loss now.

Teaching People How to Treat You

We really do teach people how to treat us. Instead of simply complaining about how people treat you, it is time to learn how to renegotiate your relationships to have what you want. You teach people to treat you well with dignity and respect, or you do not. It is as simple as that. This means you are partly responsible for the mistreatment you receive at the hands of someone else. You actually shape other people's behavior when you teach them what they can or cannot get away with.

If the people in your life are treating you poorly, figure out what you might be doing to allow, elicit or reinforce that treatment. What are the payoffs for that person when they treat you poorly? For example, when people are being controlling, and they get their way, you have rewarded them for unacceptable behavior.

You can negotiate a new relationship with that person, but you must do so from a position of power and strength, not self-doubt or fear. Resolve to be treated with dignity and respect that is uncompromised. The worst thing you could do is make a lot of noise about resetting only to revert back to old, unhealthy habits. If you talk about making changes and you do not do it yourself, you are teaching that person to take what you say lightly.

Commit to your health. Commit to yourself, although it make be difficult at times to make effective changes. You must not compromise. To compromise in the area of your health is to sell out your most precious commodity — YOU.

Breaking Up With Food as a Relationship

It may take a while for the tiny voice in your head to strengthen and override those unreasonable fears of food and fat, for example, that you have tried to control for so long. Your desire to change and be healthy is the first step toward having the courage to keep moving forward. You may understand your "emotional" eating and discovered you are not a bad person. The choices you were making may have worked for you, but at a price, you realized, was too high to pay. You now realize you can make food choices that work better for you.

You can now see you can have a happy, satisfying life without having a love relationship with food. You are stronger and have shifted away from wanting food all the time out of respect for yourself. When you realize how much food has meant to you over the years, and how much you can use it for your health benefits, you can give permission for it to leave you. You know you will be okay. As you continue to lose weight, you will notice cravings will go away and you can experience a peace you may have not felt for years, if ever.

Of course, you still need to eat. That's the trickiest part. You need food to live and it's everywhere. You might be wondering how you can keep a former love interest of food around without dangerously embracing bad or unhealthy foods. You might be at risk of overeating and getting heavy again. Of course you are going to think about food, especially when you are hungry. You need to understand you are in a process of growing out of a powerful, compelling lifetime habit. You need to relax and give yourself some time to adjust to what has proven to be a lasting and real change in your relationship with food.

Guilt

It may be one thing when you are 10 years old and experience guilt when your mother catches you in the cookie jar before dinner. However, it is another thing when you have guilt as an adult from eating Häagen-Dazs ice cream after a long day at work or refilling your wine glass. Guilt after eating can be quite damaging to your psyche, and it is quite common, especially among health-conscious women.

Guilt can happen when you have been really good about eating healthy and exercising regularly, and then you eat a chocolate-chip cookie. You might get really upset with yourself and feel like you have totally sabotaged your weight loss efforts. Why can't we give ourselves a break? It does not help matters when everywhere you look you see magazines and billboards touting guilt-free desserts, snacks and burgers. Their underlying message is clear: if the foods pictured are guilt-free, then the other versions you are eating are guilt-ridden.

However, guilt goes much deeper than that. It can come from feeling that we always need to be perfect. In other words, making healthy food choices becomes a performance of "being good." We want to prove that we are excelling at eating healthy and capable of succeeding at losing weight and keeping it off. It can be tricky. Many people deny their body food based on what they think is right. This can make you choose the "wrong" pleasure foods, which in turn makes us feel guilty instead of satisfied. How do you stop those food-induced guilt trips?

Before social media, we were exposed to celebrities with perfect bodies on billboards, television, movies, and magazines. Now, with social media, we are blasted with these types of images all the time. It can be quite damaging trying to live up to that perfect image, making comparisons and in constant scrutiny of our own body. You may have noticed you receive positive attention for losing weight.

We end up relying on other people's judgment of ourselves for a standard of comparison. Tweets and comments may seem innocent or simple, but they can really have an impact in a negative way causing unrealistic expectations about what "thin" is. On the other hand, you can use the Internet for support and inspiration, and as a powerful tool for recovery and health, not guilt.

EFFECTS PHARMACEUTICAL COMPANIES HAVE ON OUR WEIGHT

Wouldn't it be wonderful if we could simply take a pill and lose weight? There are endless pharmaceutical companies used in weight loss therapy such as those that reduce your appetite and stimulate the central nervous system. Others increase levels of serotonin in the brain, helping you feel full or prevent fat absorption in the gut from occurring. Regardless of how these drugs work, they only help you lose weight if you limit your caloric intake.

The side effects of these weight loss drugs may be rather extensive and include:

- Hypertension (high blood pressure)
- Heart disease
- Increased pulse and heart rate
- Restlessness
- Dizziness
- Insomnia
- Dry mouth
- Constipation
- Headache
- Runny nose
- Sore throat
- Diarrhea
- Oily stools
- Gas
- Decrease in absorption of fat-soluble vitamins

Using weight loss medications may result in abuse and dependence. Other side effects may include personality changes, irritability, psychosis, and severe insomnia. Driving a car may be more difficult when on these medications. Difficulty breathing, chest pain, edema and fainting may also occur. If you already have any kind of medical condition, high blood pressure or diabetes, you must talk to your doctor before considering taking medication. High doses can result in hallucinations; toxic psychosis is also possible with excessive or even proper use.

Some weight loss drugs can also increase the risk for kidney and gallbladder stones. There are many over-the-counter diet pills approved for weight loss and prevent absorption of ingested fat from being stored in the body. However, the side effects are just as unpleasant; they include oily stools, discharge and potential bowel accidents if you eat too much fat at a meal and take the product.

Many over-the-counter diet supplements are promoted as helping with weight loss, but few are proven to work. In fact, some of the ingredients may be downright dangerous. The FDA classifies herbal products as dietary supplements, meaning they are unregulated and can be marketed without the years of testing and regulatory review required by prescription and non-prescription drugs. Here are some common ingredients seen in over-the-counter diet supplements:

Hydroxycitric acid — Derived from the fruit of a tree native to Southeast Asia; however, it has been shown to cause cardiovascular disorders, serious muscle damage, and seizures.

Green Tea Extract — Can cause liver problems in concentrated forms; it should be consumed as a tea.

Chromium — A mineral you can get through your diet in meats, whole grains, and some fruits and vegetables. It has been linked to headaches and dizziness.

Conjugated linoleic acid (CLA) — Found naturally in dairy and meat products and may cause stomach upset.

Chitosan — Made from the starch found in shellfish.

Pyruvate — Produced by the body as a result of the breakdown of protein and carbohydrate found in wine, red apples, and cheese.

St. John's Wort — An herb that works as an anti-depressant — but can interact with out drugs.

Aloe — Can lead to mineral depletion or ulcerative colitis, especially if you have pre-existing intestinal issues.

Cascara — Interacts with other drugs and throws off the body's mineral balance.

Guarana — Can increase blood pressure. It should be avoided at all costs.

Yerba Mate — Often used as a tea, and can result in overstimulation of the central nervous system and high blood pressure.

Guar Gum — Used as a thickening agent in many commercially-made foods, but when taken alone can swell on contact with liquid.

Ma Huang or **Ephedra** — The FDA banned its sale from dietary supplements in 2004. It can cause cardiovascular problems including high blood pressure.

DO YOU UNDERSTAND YOUR BODY?

Understanding your body is a foreign concept to many people. We are simply unaware of what our body movements and posture mean. Think about an animal you approach that cowers when you go to pet them. You know immediately that they have been through some sort of abuse mentally or physically. The same goes for us. If we grow up in a healthy environment, we develop a healthy, happy body that moves with ease and grace. The opposite is true for those who grow up in a dangerous environment. They learn how to hide their fear and do whatever they need to survive. If a person's spirit is broken, their head may hang down and shoulders droop, developing a humpback over time. My point is that it is important to understand your body's posture. It is the first step toward mind-body healing and having body self-awareness.

As someone who has been in the fitness world my whole life, I enjoy looking at the posture of my clients and try to understand their life story. It can tell me a lot about what is happening on the inside. You can do it too. Look around you at people wherever you are and do a posture analysis of them. Do they hold their body upright in an easy, neutral position? Do they stand like a soldier at attention? Are they slumped forward? Do they have trouble standing or sitting still? Do they look calm or appear anxious? Very few people have self-awareness of their body.

Body movements and postures are very telling signs your body is giving in to the stresses of the world. All of these various non-neutral postures can take their toll over time. Understanding your body will help you understand your body, mind, and soul issues. When you have self-awareness of your body, you can take the next step: give your body what it needs to heal and run at optimum levels. Your body needs sound nutrition, regular exercise and time to quiet your mind and soul.

Exercise: How Much Do You Really Need?

For many people, finding the time to exercise can be a struggle, but you may be overestimating how much exercise you really need. Spending hours in the gym is not the answer for most people. It simply is not realistic. Short, frequent bouts of exercise can still yield results, especially when combined with healthy meals. For example, the American Journal of Sports Medicine published a study showing short walks after dinner were very effective in reducing body fat and lowering blood pressure and triglyceride levels, in addition to weight loss.

Let's face it — everyone can find five minutes to devote to exercise a few times per day. Use the time to exercise while waiting in line at the grocery store by doing side leg lifts, for example, or if you are sitting in a chair with your laptop computer, practice leg lifts and squeeze your quadriceps with each lift. Increasing the intensity in short increments can really work for keeping you in the fitness mindset. Of course, the goal should be longer workouts on a consistent basis; this is crucial to optimum health and vitality.

Good health really comes from doing at least 30 minutes of physical activity at least 5 days per week. It takes about 5 minutes to begin to feel the endorphin rush that comes with doing exercise. Choose activities that work several large muscle groups at once or using exercises engaging more than one body part at a time are really most effective. For example, you can practice doing 5 minutes of squats while lifting your arms in front of you such as standing and almost sitting down in a chair. It is amazing how quickly your body adapts to an exercise so it is important to change your exercises and routines from time to time to keep your body guessing.

Add jumping jacks to the mix or if you take a walk on a daily basis, try walking backwards (if it is safe to do so) or zigzag your walking. Pick up speed or walk for 2 minutes and run for 1 minute to continue to gain benefits form shorts bursts of activity. If you can't meet with your personal trainer (me) then you might feel a bit guilty and it is still important to get that walk in. Keep your eye on the prize — meaning how much better you look and healthier you feel.

Time Management Tips

If I had a dollar for every time I heard from someone they do not have any time to exercise, I would be extremely wealthy. However, it usually is not a lack of time but more a lack of enjoying exercise, lack of motivation, or a negative connotation about exercise such as "it is going to hurt" or "I will be sore." As busy as we all are, we all seem to find time to work on our computer or watch television. We may all have a good reason but it really comes down to time management.

Think about what will happen down the road if you ignore your health or exercise habits. Would you like to spend time in the doctor's office? Will you have the time and money to take medication for high blood pressure or another illness or disease? If you want to exercise, you will find the time. Here are some smart strategies for making exercise a part of your life:

Figure Out the Best Time For YOU To Exercise — Make it a part of your calendar. Schedule it. Work your life around your exercise plan. It will help you stay motivated and help you do something for yourself.

Consider Trading 30 Minutes Of TV Time For Exercise — Before you sit down on the couch, consider doing some form of exercise. If you must watch television, do some push-ups, lunges, yoga poses, or planks. Be old-school and watch some commercials! Use the commercial time to do some jumping jacks or run in place.

Change Your Thought Patterns — Instead of saying, "I don't have time to exercise," think "I do have time for myself and my health." Make yourself a priority.

Share Exercise With Your Partner — Take a yoga class together or salsa lessons. Go on a hike or plan a picnic with healthy foods.

Work Exercise In With A Friend — Instead of meeting for lunch or dinner, go for a leisurely bike ride or meet for a yoga or Zumba class at your local gym.

Get Creative With Exercise — In other words, exercise wherever you are. For example, while standing at the kitchen sink, do calf raises. Perform squats when picking up trash, towels or clothes off the floor. If you are a new mother, pick your baby up and do a few overhead lifts — it also should make your baby laugh. If you spend hours at soccer practice for your children, take your bicycle and ride around the field while they practice. Instead of trying to fit one more errand in while your kids are busy with their activities, take a walk.

Nominate Your Motivator — It might be a friend, family member or personal trainer (me, again) to be your cheerleader for fitness. Getting excited about fitness is contagious and you will find time to do it.

Find The Right Workout For You — Part of staying motivated and finding time to exercise is choosing an exercise program that fits your personality. Look for something you enjoy doing and actually look forward to doing.

Make Exercise A Part Of Family Life — Schedule after-dinner walks, family trips to the gym, or bike rides. It will set a good example to your children making them realize exercise is important.

Plan For Travel — Invest in an exercise band that fits easily in any suitcase. Pack your workout clothes and plan on using the fitness facility at your hotel.

Do "Something" On the Hour — Many of us spend long hours on the computer. Make a point of getting up on the hour and going for a 10-minute walk, put in a DVD and do a yoga or Pilates workout or do random sets of weightlifting with a set of dumbbells. Do a 90-second workout with 30 seconds of push-ups, 30 seconds of holding the plank position, and 30 seconds of squats or alternating lunges.

Get A Pedometer — It will really surprise you when you realize how much you are walking. Aim for at least 10,000 steps per day. Climbing a flight of stairs is equivalent to 100 steps.

Metabolism

Your body may not be burning calories quickly enough due to poor eating habits and a sedentary lifestyle. Fortunately, you can boost your metabolism and rev up your inner engine to lose weight with more energy. If your body's engine is running at full-speed, there's little you can do to boost your fat-burning potential — you're already performing at peak. But if your tank is teetering on half-empty, there's room for improvement. Use these 7 FITamentalist tips to rev up your metabolism:

FITamentalist Tip #1: Get To Bed Early

Getting enough hours of sleep can have a big effect on your waistline. Studies show sleep deprivation can send your hunger and appetite hormones out of whack. Make a point of shutting down the computer around 9:00 p.m. Turn the lights down lower and aim for a 10:00 p.m. bedtime, especially if you have to get up at an early hour.

FITamentalist Tip #2: Get Up Earlier

Does your morning ritual consist of showering, brushing your teeth, and getting dressed? Then you're neglecting two important activities that could boost your metabolism. The first one is eating breakfast — and just drinking coffee doesn't count. Skipping that bowl of oatmeal might sound harmless, but you're missing the first opportunity of the day to jumpstart your metabolism.

Secondly, you should exercise. Sure, you might struggle to throw off those cozy sheets, but it's a battle worth winning. Why? It boosts your metabolism. You'll burn more calories throughout the day simply doing the same stuff you always do. Even a 20-minute walk or jog will make a difference. So skip that second cup of java and strap on your walking shoes instead.

FITamentalist Tip #3: Make An Effort To Move More

It may sound impossible, but you can — and should — exercise every day. Exercise stimulates your metabolism and helps burn calories that can even temporarily suppress your appetite post-workout. The program will boost lean muscle tissue mass that will enable you to burn more calories per pound than fat. The more lean muscle tissue you have, the more calories you burn daily.

FITamentalist Tip #4: Eat Mini-Meals Every 3-4 Hours

Forget about three large square meals a day. Graze on healthy snacks or nosh on smaller meals instead. Eating 5-6 small meals throughout the day keeps a steady stream of energy available to your body that will boost your metabolism as well as brainpower. Keep healthy snacks (fruits, veggies, yogurt and nuts) with you throughout the day. Just be sure your main meals are smaller to accommodate all this snacking, or you'll load up on extra calories you don't need.

Do NOT skip meals. Dieters often try to get that extra weight-loss edge by cutting entire meals instead of just cutting calories throughout the day. This is counterproductive: skipping meals forces your metabolism to slow down and conserve calories to compensate for the lack of food plus it will be more difficult for you to do your workout if you are not properly fueled.

FITamentalist Tip #5: Raise A Glass (Of Water)

The number on the scale may look good when you haven't had enough water, but you're risking major weight gain by not drinking enough. Dehydration can trick your brain into thinking you're hungry, so instead of reaching for a cold one — water, that is — you reach for whatever snack is nearby. Make sure you are drinking enough water throughout the day.

FITamentalist Tip #6: Eat Spicy Foods

Turning up the heat on your meals may do more than just add fun flavor. "Hot" foods, such as jalapeños, chili peppers and spices (like curry and cayenne), may increase body temperature. Body temperature and metabolism are related: as you burn energy, heat is released. By increasing your internal body temperature, spicy foods may temporarily raise your metabolism and stimulate the use of stored fat as energy. If you are not a fan of spicy foods, experiment with different vinegars or milder spices such as cinnamon, nutmeg, or herbs to add flavor and just a little bit of heat.

FITamentalist Tip #7: Count On Calcium

Look for a good quality calcium/magnesium supplement to take at night about an hour before bed. Calcium and magnesium should be in a 2:1 ratio such as 500 mg of calcium with 250 mg of magnesium. It helps lower blood pressure by relaxing the muscles including your heart for a great night's sleep so you are raring to go in the morning.

Understanding and Respecting Exercise Benefits

The benefits of exercise are endless, whether it is cardiovascular fitness, building muscle, or achieving gains in strength. Bodyweight exercises need to be a part of your workout regimen. Combining cardiovascular workouts with strength training makes for one quick workout that will keep your heart pumping while encouraging the growth of muscle and strength. One of the best benefits of exercise is it still is the best way to lose weight. There are no shortcuts, and exercise has a major impact your metabolism.

Regardless of your fitness level, it is never too late to start. Performing an exercise super slow or a little faster, perhaps adding extra repetitions can make the simplest exercise a bit more challenging. When it comes to your core, know that it is more than your abdominal muscles. Your core is made up of 29 muscles, and many exercises can engage all of them. A strong core equals improved performance in any activity, as well as better posture.

One of the best things you can do for yourself as you exercise is maintain flexibility. Being able to perform an exercise with a full range of motion can reduce the chance of injury and lead to improved posture. Yoga is an excellent way to improve strength while improving flexibility plus a regular practice helps you connect to your inner being. If you are new to yoga, come to your mat with an open mind and heart, without any expectations. When you don't have any expectations, you can experience immense joy.

Before You Say "It Is Inconvenient To Exercise"

Before you say it is inconvenient to exercise or you don't have any time, you can still squeeze in a workout any time of day, no matter where you are. Exercising without equipment can be a huge stress reliever whether you are at home or on the road. Having no time is not an excuse. Exercise can also give you better balance increasing control and body awareness.

Keep exercise interesting. Head outdoors and use the equipment in your local park for a workout. Practice yoga outside on a beautiful day. There are countless ways to add variation to your workout routine. Staying fit can be fun and enjoyable. Regular exercise can actually help you stay pain-free, one of the best benefits of all. If you are new to weight training, it always ideal to me with a personal trainer (me) and learn proper form and technique.

Injury Prevention

Now that you have committed to getting in shape, you are probably eager to see results. Be patient. Moving ahead too fast can lead to injuries. In some cases, doing a particular exercise using the wrong form or technique can cause an injury. Perhaps you might be doing the same exercise too often. Here are some tips that will help you avoid fitness injuries and workout smart:

Know Your Body's Limitations — This means knowing any weak areas or avoiding activities that might push you too hard. For example, if you have had knee or hip surgery, you might be more comfortable on a stationary bike as opposed to a treadmill. Avoid activities that cause pain.

Take Precautions When You Exercise — For example, women tend to be more flexible and do well with yoga, Pilates, cycling, or stepping, while men do well with restricted formats such as weight lifting.

Hire A Professional — Taking sessions with a professional, certified trainer, like myself, will ensure your body is in proper alignment during your exercise routine, motivate you to continue your exercise program, and help you prevent any injuries. A personal trainer can give you an appropriate workout routine, suggest the right amount of weight to lift and give you time to rest (but not too long). The right exercise program will allow your muscles to heal and avoid injury.

Athletic Dreams Die Hard — It is important to perform exercises appropriate for your age. Doing too much too quickly or with too much intensity can lead to an injury. A personal trainer can ensure you are doing the right exercises for your age.

Warming Up IS Necessary — Regardless of the exercises you are going to perform, warming up will go a long way in preventing an injury. Warming up helps your muscles handle the stress of the workout and decreases the risk of injury. If you are lifting weights, you can start with lighter weights and do 20 repetitions to warm up that specific muscle group.

Slowly Build Up The Pace Of Your Workout — If you are just beginning, start with the amount of weight that allows you to perform at least 10-12 repetitions. Overestimating your strength can lead to improper form and technique, and increases the risk for injury. Moderation is key.

Vary Your Workouts — This is an excellent way to prevent injuries because you will not repeat the same muscle movements which can lead to overuse and repetitive-use injuries. For example, ride your bicycle one day and lift weights the next day. Give your muscles time to rest and recover, especially if you are sore.

Heart Rate

Knowing your target heart rate is the simplest way to know if you are overdoing it or not working hard enough. In other words, you do not want to over-exercise nor should you lack exercise. Before you figure out your target training heart rate, you must know your resting heart rate. Your resting heart rate is the number of times your heart beats in one minute while at rest. Before you get out of bed in the morning, you can check your resting heart rate by placing your fingers on your ceratoid artery in your neck or use your wrist. Count how many times your pulse is beating for one minute.

Average Resting Heart Rates:
Children 10 years old – adults (including seniors) = 60-100 beats per minute (bpm)
Well-trained athletes = 40-60 bpm

Target Training Heart Rate:
Take your pulse on the inside of your wrist using the first two fingers and press lightly over the blood vessels on your wrist. Count your pulse for 10 seconds and multiply by 6 = your bpm
You should stay between 50% and 85% of your maximum heart rate for your target heart rate.

220 – Age = Maximum Heart Rate

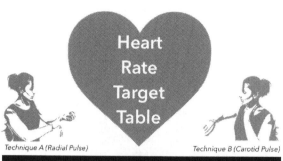

Technique A (Radial Pulse)　　　　　　　　　　Technique B (Carotid Pulse)

30 Second Calculation (Using either Technique A (Radial Pulse) inside the wrist (below the thumb joint) or Technique B (Carotid Pulse) on the neck at the side of the windpipe.					
Age	55%	60%	70%	80%	85%
15	19	21	24	27	29
20	18	20	23	27	28
25	18	19	23	26	28
30	17	19	22	25	27
35	17	19	22	25	26
40	17	18	21	24	26
45	16	18	20	23	25
50	16	17	20	23	24
55	15	17	19	22	23
60	15	16	19	21	23
65	14	16	18	21	22
70	14	15	18	20	21
75	13	15	17	19	21
80	13	14	16	19	20

Using the target heart rate chart above, you can find your age and what your target heart rate should be. During moderately intense exercise, it should be 50-69% of your maximum heart rate whereas your heart rate during a hard workout is about 70% to less than 90% of the maximum heart rate. Keep in mind that blood pressure medications lower maximum heart rates and can also change your target heart rate zone.

What Does This All Mean?

If you are straining and your heart rate is too high, slow down. If the intensity of your exercise feels easy or moderate you may want to push yourself a bit more. If you are a beginner, aim for a lower range of your target zone at first and gradually build up to a higher range. You will eventually be able to comfortably exercise at 85% of your maximum heart rate. A good rule of thumb is you should be able to carry on a conversation while exercising. If not, you might be doing too much.

If you are dealing with any sort of heart condition, you should have permission from your physician to engage in an exercise program. He or she may recommend that you train with a personal trainer to ensure you are being monitored during exercise. Plus, a personal trainer can choose exercises appropriate for your condition and current fitness level.

Cortisol and Stress (Liquid Pounds)

You may have heard an advertisement on television or radio about cortisol and how by reducing it you can achieve successful weight loss. However, cortisol is a hormone produced by the adrenal glands. Its main function is to increase the flow of protein, fat and glucose out of your tissues and into circulation. Cortisol levels are highest in the morning when you first wake up and peak about 30 minutes later before declining throughout the day. Cortisol is also released in response to emotional and physical stress.

At the right times and in the right amount, cortisol offers many benefits anyone wanting to lose body fat and keep muscle. Cortisol does not cause inflammation, but it does increase in response to inflammation. This helps repair muscle damage after a workout, which is why supplements that block cortisol are not a good idea. Cortisol actually increases the rate at which stored body fat is released from the fat cells. However, if cortisol levels are raised for long periods of time, it is often due to psychological or physiological stress such as eating too few calories or exercising excessively.

One of the issues with high cortisol levels is water retention. When you lift weights, the body sends water to surround the muscle tissue that has been torn down. The extra water can appear like you have not lost any body fat. In other words, the number of the scale remains the same. When you train hard, you release a lot of cortisol and it can make your body appear puffy or bloated. Healthy food and rest are the main things that stop cortisol once it is increased.

I have seen dieters and athletes increase ten pounds simply by doing extreme workouts without carbohydrates. That increase in bloating or retention of water makes you look different. It may look like fat, but it isn't. That is why some people lose weight quickly when they "cheat." Retained water and cortisol levels drop and they look several pounds lighter. An increase in cortisol for a prolonged period of time is not good for your muscles. Cortisol:

1. Prevents protein synthesis
2. Promotes the breakdown of protein
3. Counters the effects of other anabolic hormones including testosterone

Cortisol does not cause weight gain, but it does make your brain less sensitive to the effects of leptin. Leptin is a hormone that signals satiety, and cortisol can dull that signal and leave you feeling hungrier than normal. It can stimulate your appetite, particularly for foods that are high in sugar, fat, and starch. When we are stressed, this problem can be made worse with large amounts of cortisol being secreted, which is why some people turn to food and eat more when they are stressed out; high-fat foods, sugar, and starch calm the body's response to stress.

We do not all respond to stress in the same way, so when the source of stress is removed, cortisol levels will return to normal at different speeds. Some people lose weight when they are stressed simply because they eat less food. However, more people tend to eat more food in response to stress. Recognizing when you are stressed is the first step in addressing the issue and how best to handle it that works for you.

Hydration

Water is necessary for every process in the body. When you think about that, you realize how much your body depends on water for survival. Every organ, tissue, and cell needs water to work properly. Water is needed for good health and for your body to lubricate the joints, maintain temperature, and remove toxins and waste.

You lose water every day through simply breathing, sweating, going to the bathroom, and when you exercise. If you do not replace the water lost, you can become dehydrated. If you experience any of the following symptoms, you may be dehydrated:

1. Headache
2. Dizziness
3. Fatigue
4. Confusion
5. Dry mouth or extreme thirst
6. Dark urine

The first thing you should do upon waking up is to drink some water. Starting your day with water is an excellent way to hydrate the body before that morning cup of coffee. Coffee dehydrates the body, so you are already at a deficit upon waking. Drinking plenty of water throughout the day is a great way to actively prevent dehydration. You might need to increase your water intake if you are:

- Pregnant
- Breastfeeding
- Exercising
- Trying to lose weight
- Outside in hot weather
- Dealing with a medical condition such as a bladder infection or kidney stones

You have probably heard the recommendation to drink 6-8 eight-ounce glasses of water per day, and that is definitely doable. Some people need a little bit less while others need more. One of the best ways to tell if you are not drinking enough water is if your urine is a dark amber or dark yellow color. If your urine is light yellow or colorless, you are well hydrated.

Stay away from soft drinks to stay hydrated as they often add extra sugar and calories to your diet. Who needs that? Besides, your body wants the water, not a sugary soft drink. Fruit and vegetable juices, herbal teas, coffee, and milk can contribute to your daily water intake. However, watch the caffeine intake, as that can make you urinate more frequently or make you feel nervous or anxious. Water can also be found in soup broths, fruits, and vegetables.

When it comes to sport drinks, they can increase your energy levels and help the body absorb water. They can be helpful if you are planning on exercising for longer than an hour or exercising at a high intensity. Be aware they often contain added sugar, high levels of sodium and are high in calories. Sport drinks are NOT the same as energy drinks. Energy drinks are usually full of stimulants like taurine, ginseng or guarana as well as large amounts of caffeine and sugar. Teens and children should NOT have energy drinks.

Here are some tips for staying hydrated:
- Invest in a good water bottle that you can fill up with water and ice.
- Jazz it up with a squeeze of lemon or lime
- Drink water before, during, and after your workout
- If you feel hungry, drink water first

- Drink water on the hour
- Automatically order water at a restaurant

Salt and Flavoring Alternatives

Salt has long been used as a flavor enhancer and preserver of food. Sodium actually plays an important role in maintaining blood pressure, electrolyte balance, and the body's hydration levels. In fact, there are some health benefits of "true salts," such as Himalayan Pink Salt, which are full of important minerals and will not elevate blood pressure.

Iodized salt from the salt shaker is what can really elevate blood pressure and cause inflammation, and should be avoided by anyone dealing with a health condition such as high blood pressure. However, no one should overdo it when it comes to salt. There are alternatives that add flavor to food without using salt. Here are some nutritious swap outs for salt:

Kelp Granules — Are from the sea and full of vitamins and minerals including B-vitamins, calcium, magnesium and iodine.

Liquid Aminos — Are a soy sauce alternative that is delicious on vegetables and stir-fries, and contain 16 essential amino acids and just 160 mg of sodium.

Herbs And Spices — Experiment with different herbs and spices for endless combinations that add variety and flavor. Some of my favorite herbs to use are sage, onion and garlic powder, rosemary, thyme, and oregano.

Nutritional Yeast — Serves up a savory, rich "cheesy" flavor that works well over rice, quinoa, or popcorn and can be added to sauces for an excellent substitute for salt.

CLIENT STORY: SHARON

When I work with people I ask a ton of questions, but there are three main questions I often ask:

1. What's your goal weight?
2. Name an age or time in your life you were the happiest mentally and physically.

3. How old were you when you had your first sexual experience?

This may seem like prying to some, and if I have a read on a person that they are not ready to fill me in on every part of their life and/or not emotionally stable to go there, I wait it out — but over time it is important to address these topics.

I have been a lifestyle coach and FITamentalist for over a decade. I have trained every age, gender, body size and walk of life out there. Over 35% of the clients I have trained have suffered from severe PTSD at one time or another, whether they know it or not. At least 30% of those clients were sexually abused as children or violated sexually in their adulthood. According to the Centers for Disease Control and Prevention's ACE Study, more than six million obese and morbidly obese people are likely to have suffered physical, sexual, and/or verbal abuse during their childhoods.

Sharon was referred to me by a massage therapist with whom I used to work and to whom I continue to refer my clients. Sharon was 5'5" and weighed around 190 pounds. Sharon used to be a competitive bodybuilder, competing for over a decade, but her weight would constantly fluctuate depending on the next show. When Sharon competed, she would weigh in at 150 pounds with 3-5% body fat. Off-season, she would balloon to over 200 pounds. Over the years, Sharon won numerous titles while working full time as a legal assistant.

Sharon was soft-spoken and though her frame was massive and intimidating when she competed, she was really childlike when you got to know her. As I have noticed with a lot of competitors, when they leave competing they can get lost and have a hard time adapting to the reset of eating and being a non-competitor. Competitors are great at knowing how to starve themselves and have no life in season, and pig out with the worst foods out there in the off-season.

Sharon, being out of competition for a few years at this point, had trouble staying motivated and finding activities that made the workout fun. For over a decade, competing was her life, her fall-back career, and her perfect excuse to be as anti-social as she wanted. Women who body-build are fascinating and highly respected, in my eyes. I get why men like to be massive and work out with the testosterone they have, but I never really understoond why it would be appealing for a woman to compete.

After working with Sharon for a few months I felt comfortable enough with her to discuss her competition days and what got her into it. Sharon came right out and told me that from the age of three to seven years of age, her grandfather molested her. Until she started therapy, she never told a soul — not even her husband. Until her divorce 3 years ago, she didn't realize the trauma she suppressed led her to every choice she made in her life, without even realizing it. She never had children because she believed she couldn't trust anyone around them. She married a kind and decent man but cheated on him many times because she didn't feel worthy of his love and sabotaged the relationship.

She held on to the shame, pain, and secrets; her grandfather's abuse left her feeling horrible inside, and, according to her, she never let anyone in. The divorce and the depression of it all left her no choice but to check into an extensive therapy program that forced her to confront the past and stop holding onto her grandfather's shame. Before entering therapy, Sharon never told any friends, teachers, her husband, or even her mother about the abuse she dealt with as a child. She didn't want to tell her mother because her whole life, her mother suffered from alcoholism and clinical depression.

Sharon never wanted to be a burden, so she took it into her own hands and became her own protector. Instead of turning to food for comfort, she found control by having a perfect body. She built a massive protective shield of muscle that made her feel powerful and safe. She promised to never be powerless again, the way she'd felt as a vulnerable child — taken advantage of. Her emotions might have been scarred, but she would be damned if it reflected on the outside.

EXCUSE #8:
IF I LIFT WEIGHTS, I WILL LOOK LIKE A BODYBUILDER

By this week, if you have been following the strength-training component of *The Reset Plan*, you should be starting to see improved muscle definition and increased strength. Many women become fearful about where this is going to end if they stick with a weight-training program. This chapter discusses myths and benefits of continued weight training and strategies for controlling how and where we build muscle.

This chapter confronts two very common excuses people make to keep from exercising, but it really addresses the importance of building a community that will be supportive of your fitness goals and commitment to a healthy lifestyle. It also offers practical guidance for those who want to work out at home. You will also be guided through specific cardio and strength training "upgrades" this week, as well as challenged to begin making even healthier choices regarding protein within the parameters of their food plan.

VISUALIZATION

You may have convinced yourself that genetically, you were never meant to be built like Sophia Loren, Jennifer Lopez, or whomever you may admire these days, but you need to know it is just as tough for them to keep their amazing physiques. There is no doubt in my mind they use visualization and imagery to gain muscle, slim down, and focus on their fitness goals. Visualization means having a clear picture in your mind of what you want to achieve. It helps trigger positive emotions, supports your ability to make smart decisions and make any corrections in your eating habits and exercise program as needed.

Visualization takes concentration, mindfulness, and focused effort deep inside of you. The objective is to improve your non-judgmental awareness of your body's emotions and sensations. Mindfulness is like creating a movie in your head about what you want to look like. You can be as specific as you like. It means taking the time to slow down, sit quietly and turn inward so you can assess your emotions, thoughts and feelings. Yes, we are talking about meditation, and it allows you be totally involved and immersed in whatever activity you are doing.

The process can help get your muscles to respond to what you want them to do. Take some time to go within and watch all the sensations you are feeling — no judgment. You have the potential to dramatically change the shape of your body and the way your body responds to exercise, especially when you do it without judgment.

Visualization is the ability to create vivid images in your mind of a desired outcome. You can actually reprogram your subconscious mind, the part of the brain that processes thoughts and decisions, and trigger emotions. By visualizing positive outcomes, you can turn your dream into a reality. Here are the steps to follow when learning to visualize:

Step 1: Create The Image In Your Mind

Be specific as possible. Look at images of the guy or the girl you physically would like to *Reset* to look like. Without comparing yourself to them, put on your appreciation glasses and check in with what about them appeals to you? What have they reset or worked hard to achieve that you haven't and may be lacking? Maybe the person has washboard abs or tight glutes. Use these images to create the mental image in your mind of what you want to achieve. Look in the mirror and envision the body that you want looking back at you. Be realistic.

Step 2: Concentrate And Learn To Meditate

Using visualization requires concentration, focus and mindfulness. This is more commonly known as meditation. The foundation of meditation is mindfulness. Pay attention to the present moment without judgment. It is all about quieting your mind. If thoughts come in, let them come in and take a deep breath in and let them go right where you are. When you take some time to meditate, you become better able to improve your thought patterns, regulate emotions, improve relationships with others and bodily functions.

When you practice mindfulness, it allows you to totally immerse yourself into your workout that will give you that extra edge to reach the next level. It can help you get in touch with your muscles to make them work for you, not against you.

Step 3: Before You Go To The Gym

Before you go to the gym, take about 10 minutes to sit quietly in a room without any distractions. Close your eyes and focus on your breath as you go within. Let your body relax and allow the image in your mind of what you want to achieve to flow into your mind. Get a clear picture of your desired physique. Then, focus on what you are going to do during your workout that day. Imagine performing each exercise with perfect form and control. Take a moment to feel your muscles contracting, and the confidence and satisfaction you feel when you see your muscles flex in the mirror.

If a negative thought comes in, change it or reverse it. Keep your thoughts positive. Always end your meditation practice on a positive note. These positive thoughts will ignite your passion for working out so you can perform at your best.

Step 4: Practice Makes Perfect

Visualization takes practice and should be done daily. Eventually, you will be able to concentrate on your vision and control your thoughts. You must make an effort to make your mental images of what you want to achieve a reality. Creating a lean, sculpted body takes hard work and visualization is just one part.

Visualization can enhance your overall attitude and enhance performance in the gym. Practicing the techniques, strategies and eating plans in this book will help you train like a champion. Perform your workouts with intensity and enthusiasm. Be honest with yourself. You are ready for the journey.

MUSCLE MYTHS AND FACTS

There is so much information out there about what to eat, how long to rest, and what exercises are required to build a lean physique. It is time to dispel the myths and set you straight with the facts about muscle. Let's start with the myths about muscle:

Myth #1: You Have To Eat A Huge Amount Of Protein To Build Muscle

While you need the right amount of protein per day for muscle growth, in general, the amount required is nowhere near as much as most people think. Athletes need 2 grams of protein per body weight of total protein per day to optimize protein synthesis and muscle growth in the body.

Myth #2: Supplementing With Protein Powder Is More Effective In Building Muscle

There is no evidence that supplementing with protein powder is more effective for muscle growth than protein found in food. They are quite expensive and you can choose good quality protein found in food such as eggs or lean meats like chicken and fish, which all provide a wide range of amino acids. Protein powder is processed no matter how you look at it.

Do you like chocolate milk? Well, the good news is drinking low-fat chocolate milk after a workout can help build muscle and endurance, reduces fat, and seems to improve performance. Low-fat chocolate milk has the right combination of protein and carbohydrates. When you are recovering from your workout, you want to turn on protein synthesis and stop the breakdown of protein. Plus, you want to replenish sugar stores in the muscle; the combination of proteins and carbohydrates work together in chocolate milk to help you recover from your workout. (Journal of Nutrition and Metabolism)

Myth #3: You Need To Perform 3 Sets Of 15 Repetitions To Gain Muscle

You may think doing more repetitions is more effective in synthesizing protein in the body and gaining muscle. However, it is now known that activating the muscle fibers is the key to increasing muscle as well as strength and is more important than the number of sets or repetitions. Many people go through the motions of doing an exercise or perform an exercise too fast. Slow and controlled movements in a set can be judged by the following: the last three repetitions should be hard to do. If they are not, it is probably time to increase the weight.

Myth #4: The More Protein You Eat After A Workout, The Greater The Muscle Growth

Although it is important to eat high quality protein after a workout, there does not seem to be a relationship between the amount of muscle gained and the amount of protein consumed. You want to consume about 20 grams of protein in the three hours after a workout and adequate protein at regular intervals throughout the day for effective muscle growth. Anything more than that will not contribute to more synthesis of muscle. I grew up thinking protein is healthy and I can have as much as I want. Protein breaks down into excess calories if you eat too much… just like anything else.

Myth #5: Carbohydrates Do Not Play A Role In Muscle Growth

Many people think protein is the key nutrient to build muscle and carbohydrates do not play a role in this process. Carbohydrates are essential fuel for muscles and they contain sugars, starches and fiber. With the exception of fiber, all carbohydrates are converted during digestion into smaller molecules of glucose, the essential source of energy used by every cell in the body. Carbohydrates are mostly plant-based foods such as fruits, vegetables, grains, and legumes.

Simple carbohydrates are all single- (monosaccharides) and double-chained sugars (disaccharides).You can recognize them because they usually end with "-ose": glucose and fructose (from fruit), lactose (from dairy), and the table sugar sucrose (from beet or cane sugar).

Simple sugars are usually added to low-fat foods to give them flavor, but they lack nutrition because they don't contain many micronutrients, vitamins, minerals or phytochemicals.

Good carbohydrates include whole grains (oats, some cereals, rye, millet, quinoa, whole wheat and brown rice), beans, legumes, fruits and vegetables. Bad carbohydrates are refined or processed foods.

Complex carbohydrates are many chains of simple sugars joined together (oligosaccharides and polysaccharides). They include starch, a form of carbohydrates plants store, and fiber, the mostly undigested part of the plant. Foods that contain complex carbs include grains, breads, pasta, beans, potatoes, corn and other vegetables.

You can find some options in the food exchange list that can increase the ability to perform resistance and strength-training exercises by providing the energy needed to complete the workout. As a result, you will have a much more effective workout. Eating protein before or after a workout and carbohydrate before and during training with plenty of water is the most effective way to build lean muscle.

Muscle FACTS

- Eat 10-20 grams of high-quality protein within the first 30 minutes after a workout for maximum muscle synthesis.

- A high-protein snack should also contain about 35 grams of good carbohydrates to maximize protein synthesis needed to build and repair muscle, and recover at a faster rate.

- Eating small amounts of high quality protein every 2-3 hours throughout the day is beneficial for muscle growth when combined with a training program.

- Milk may enhance muscle growth because it provides all the essential amino acids required for protein synthesis. Milk provides carbohydrates and high quality protein and makes an effective post workout beverage.

- In order to increase muscle mass, it is not only necessary to consume protein, but also make sure that the total amount of calories is adequate. In other words, if you are eating less calories than you need, your body may start to burn muscle for fuel, and that can cause you to lose precious muscle.

Hormones

Wouldn't it be great if we could blame everything on hormones? As a teenager, we might have blamed our acne on hormones — or, if a pregnant woman starts to cry for no reason, everyone assumes it is her hormones. It would be nice if we could blame everything on our hormones... but that is simply not realistic.

Some hormones are easy to understand, while others require a degree in science to understand how they function in the body. Here is a list of hormones you might find helpful in knowing just how they affect you:

Melatonin — Think of melatonin as your biological clock. This hormone is responsible for the way you feel throughout the day as far as alertness is concerned. Do you feel drowsy? Blame the melatonin.

Serotonin — This is the one you can blame for PMS and your moody teenager. Serotonin controls your mood, appetite, and your sleep cycles.

Thyroxin — A form of thyroid hormone, thyroxin increases the rate of your metabolism and also affects protein synthesis, which is the process that cells go through to build protein.

Epinephrine — This is one you have most likely heard of; it's also called adrenaline. Among a whole list of other things, epinephrine is responsible for what is known as the "fight-or-flight" response. This is the hormone that tells you when to fight and when it's best to run. Some of the bodily responses demonstrated when this hormone kicks in are dilated pupils, increased heart rate, and tensing of the muscles.

Norepinephrine — Also called noradrenaline, this hormone controls the heart and blood pressure. Norepinephrine also contributes to the control of sleep, arousal, and emotions. Obvious effects take place when there is too much or too little of this hormone. Too much gives you an anxious feeling while too little can leave you feeling depressed or sedated.

Dopamine — This controls the heart rate and also assists in perception; deciphering what is real and what is not.

Antimullerian Hormone — An inhibitor for the release of prolactin, the protein responsible mainly for lactation.

Adiponectin — This is a protein hormone that regulates metabolic processes such as the regulation of glucose.

Adrenocorticotropic Hormone — This assists in synthesizing corticosteroids, which are responsible for stress response, blood electrolyte levels, and other physiologic systems.

Angiotensinogen — Is responsible for the narrowing of blood vessels, a process known as vasoconstriction.

Antidiuretic Hormone — This hormone is also known by other names, but it is mainly responsible for retaining water within the kidneys.

Atrial Natriuretic Peptide — A peptide hormone secreted by the cells of the heart and other muscles, it's mostly involved with the control of water, sodium, potassium, and fat within the body.

Calcitonin — Aids in constructing bone and reducing blood calcium.

Cholecystokinin — Aids in the release of digestive enzymes for the pancreas and acts as an appetite suppressant.

Corticotrophin-Releasing Hormone — Releases cortisol in response to stress.

Erythropoietin — Stimulates the production of erythrocytes, which are blood cells responsible for delivering oxygen.

Follicle-Stimulating Hormone — Stimulates the follicles within the sex organs of both males and females.

Gastrin — Secretes gastric acid.

Ghrelin — Hunger stimulant as well as aiding in the secretion of the growth hormone.

Glucagon — Helps to increase the blood glucose level.

Growth Hormone-Releasing Hormone — As its name clearly implies, this hormone releases the growth hormone.

Human Chorionic Gonadotropin — Keeps the immune system from attacking a forming embryo during pregnancy.

Growth Hormone — Helps to stimulate growth and the reproduction of cells.

Insulin — Is responsible for several anabolic effects, primarily glucose intake.

Insulin-Like Growth Factor — Has the same effects as insulin while also regulating the growth and development of cells.

Leptin — Slows down the appetite while simultaneously speeding up metabolism.

Luteinizing Hormone — Aids ovulation in women and testosterone production in men.

Melanocyte Stimulating Hormone — Produce melanocytes, which are responsible for the pigment in skin and hair.

Orexin — Increases the appetite while also increasing your alertness and energy levels.

Oxytocin — A hormone that plays a major role in reproduction, it aids in orgasm and is also responsible for the release of breast milk.

Parathyroid Hormone — Among other functions, this hormone is mainly responsible for the activation of Vitamin D.

Prolactin — A major contributor in sexual satisfaction and the production of breast milk.

Secretin — Inhibits gastric acid production.

Aldosterone — Is mainly responsible for absorbing sodium in the kidneys to increase the volume of blood within the body.

Testosterone — The major male hormone, testosterone is responsible for sex drive, development of the sex organs, and the changes that take place during puberty.

Androstenedione — Is essentially estrogen.

Estradiol — In males, this hormone is responsible for preventing what is basically known as cell death of the germ cells. In females, this hormone is in overdrive. Among other things, estradiol accelerates height and metabolism, maintains the blood vessels and skin, aids in water retention, and even aids in hormone-sensitive cancers.

Progesterone — A major contributor to the body's support of pregnancy.

Lipotropin — Stimulates the production of pigment by aiding in melanin production.

Brain natriuretic peptide — Aids in reducing blood pressure.

Histamine — A hormone based in the stomach, histamine aids in the secreting of gastric acid.

Endothelin — Controls muscle contractions within the stomach.

Enkephalin — Is simply a pain regulator.

These are just a few examples of some of the hormones within the body; there are also more complex hormones whose functions are not easily understood. Our bodies, when in proper working order, function like well-oiled machines, and the hormones are a major part of nearly every process. Clearly, hormones are responsible for much more than angry teens, squeaky voices, and weepy pregnant women.

Genetics

We come in all shapes and sizes, light and dark, short and tall, with a wide variety of features that are pre-determined by our genetics. We can't control our traits, but when it comes to losing weight, and failing again and again, we may start to believe any exercise we do will yield less result simply because of our genetics. When it comes to weight management, we might say something like, "all the women in our family have big hips," or "our whole family is built that way."

Of course, people are built with all sorts of body types. We might label our body as pear-shaped or apple-shaped or simply carry our weight in our arms. You might add to the mix that you are athletic or not, and with all those genetic factors thrown in, you might think it is hopeless. Let's face it — everyone cannot go for a genetic test before beginning a weight loss program, and it may not matter what genetic makeup you have that could be contributing to your difficulty in losing weight.

All the research continues to show that "calories in versus calories out" is too simplistic and does not account for many real variables that have nothing to do with self-restraint or willpower. You probably already know this but it is always good to know science backs you up. You should not assume you are genetically precluded from ever being slim and healthy. It is possible to learn new behaviors with my weight management program that can be tailored to your specific needs in order to keep you at a healthy weight. Your genetic makeup doesn't have to mean you are doomed to lose the weight loss game. It just means you need a new strategy for winning at losing weight, no matter what your genetic makeup.

The Power of The Subconscious

While you may not be aware of it, your subconscious mind can and should be an excellent ally in achieving success in your life. All you have to do is establish a good working relationship with your subconscious mind. In order to do that, you must become conscious and familiar with this mysterious and interesting aspect of yourself, and the role it plays in your life. One of the best ways to do this is to say an affirmation every single day such as "my subconscious mind is my partner in my success."

We possess a second powerful mind and when we become conscious of our subconscious mind and realize it is not a figment of our imagination, the sky is the limit. We need to learn the roles and functions of each. There are two main functions of the subconscious mind; for example, the first might be "what you focus on you attract." Your subconscious mind will act upon any instruction or request you give it. Any thought repeated over and over again will make an imprint in your subconscious mind that cannot distinguish between what is real or imagined. This is why affirmations and visualizations have such a powerful effect in our lives.

You can create images in your mind and within yourself that the subconscious mind can act upon. Your conscious mind is the gatekeeper to the gates of the subconscious. It is the conscious mind's role to make sure only quality thoughts enter the subconscious. Our thoughts and beliefs will eventually manifest in our life. We must become diligent in directing and monitoring our thoughts.

Creating your own personal mind power program is like painting a blank canvas. You can become a master of your own thoughts, and life for that matter. All you have to do is be willing to put time in every single day in thinking about what you want to achieve. Each person is different and unique. It must suit your particular character and style. You might devote just twenty minutes each day that looks something like the following:

Spend 5 minutes visualizing your fitness goal.

Spend 5 minutes affirming your goal.

Spend 10 minutes on subconscious exercises for guidance.

Spend 5 minutes acknowledging your strengths and creating a success vibration.

While your goal may remain the same, the affirmations can change weekly as you make progress in your weight loss goals. You are a work in progress and your life is your canvas. Remember, what you focus on, you attract. Using your conscious and subconscious mind helps you focus on your goals.

Be Aware Of Self-Sabotaging

Have you ever wondered why you try so hard to lose weight only to sabotage your weight loss efforts? It doesn't make sense after eating healthy for days on end you would choose to order that decadent dessert or inhale a huge meal at your favorite restaurant. As the food is going down, you know you shouldn't be eating it but you can't stop yourself. I have done this myself. How does this happen? You wouldn't think one could intentionally sabotage any efforts to lose weight. What is wrong with this scenario? Even after I lost a lot of weight, I still struggled with self-sabotage.

Many times, I would chalk it up to feeling stressed out and the fact that eating comfort food made me feel better. Like you, I had to learn to recognize the pattern and train myself to make better choices. I realized the only person I was hurting was me. In other words, it was not about the food, but more about my behavior. Like any bad habit, I had to be diligent about finding another activity to do or food choice to make, and practice changing.

Self-sabotage is not healthy for anyone. When it comes to food choices, the consequences go way beyond the scale. Do not be discouraged. You can stop. If you find yourself indulging in a food for no good reason, try focusing on something else. Divert your attention to a project or another person that is life sustaining and supportive in a healthy way.

IMPORTANCE OF SLEEP AND RECOVERY FOR WEIGHT TRAINING

When you are following a weight loss program, make sure you are getting enough sleep. Sleep plays an important role in weight management. In fact, people with a lower BMI (body mass index) tend to sleep better and get plenty of shut-eye. Depriving yourself of sleep can actually cause you to gain weight. Take a look at some of the contributing factors that link weight loss with sleep:

Ghrelin and Leptin

These hormones play an important role in suppressing and stimulating your appetite. Ghrelin is released by the stomach and stimulates your appetite. Leptin is produced in the fat cells and is responsible for suppressing hunger. A lack of sleep lowers the leptin levels and increases the levels of ghrelin and that results in an increased appetite. Getting enough sleep can actually decrease your appetite and help you lose weight.

Growth Hormone

The pituitary gland secretes more growth hormones during sleep than when you are awake. Growth hormones stimulate cell reproduction, cell regeneration and cell growth. These hormones help the body build muscle, boost metabolism, and make it easier to lose weight.

Cortisol

Cortisol is known as the stress hormone. When you do not get enough sleep, cortisol levels increase while getting at least 8-9 hours of sleep lowers cortisol levels. A high level of cortisol translates to a lower metabolism. Breaking protein down into glucose is stimulated by cortisol. If you have too much glucose in the blood, the body will store it as fat. On top of that, cortisol interferes with the body's ability to build muscle. When trying to lose weight, make sure you get enough sleep and do all you can to de-stress the body to keep cortisol levels low.

Rest and Recovery

When you exercise, lift weights, or go for a run, you actually inflict small injuries to your muscles. In order to enhance your performance, you have to give your body time to heal. Sleep is when the body has a chance to recuperate. If you don't get enough sleep, you will feel tired and sluggish and that can lead to poor energy and poor eating habits. Sleeping enough hours will help your body recover, rest, and grow stronger. Sleep is a very important part of losing weight by suppressing your appetite, boosting your metabolism, and allowing your body the opportunity to rest and recover. Aim for at least 7-9 hours of sleep per night. Turn the computer off by 9:00 p.m. and turn the lights down. Set the mood for a good night's sleep.

MONSANTO

Most people associate omega-3 fatty acids with fish, but fish get them from green plants (specifically algae), which is where they all originate. Plant leaves produce these essential fatty acids ("essential" because our bodies can't produce them on their own) as part of photosynthesis.

Nutrients themselves have been around as a concept since the early 19th century, when the English doctor and chemist William Prout identified what came to be called the "macronutrients" which include protein, fat, and carbohydrates. It was thought that was pretty much all there was going on in food, until doctors noticed an adequate supply of the big three did not necessarily keep people nourished.

In nature, that is of course precisely what eating has always been: relationships among species in what we call food chains, or webs, that reach all the way down to the soil. Note that these ecological relationships are between eaters and whole foods, not nutrients. Even though the foods in question eventually get broken down in our bodies into simple nutrients, as corn is reduced to simple sugars, the qualities of the whole food are not unimportant — they govern such things as the speed at which the sugars will be released and absorbed, which we're coming to see as critical to insulin metabolism. Put another way, our bodies have a longstanding and sustainable relationship to corn we do not have to high-fructose corn syrup.

As we've shifted from leaves to seeds, the ratio of omega-6s to omega-3s in our bodies has shifted, too. At the same time, modern food-production practices have further diminished the omega-3s in our diet. Omega-3s, being less stable than omega-6s, spoil more readily, so we have selected for plants that produce fewer of them; further, when we partly hydrogenate oils to render them more stable, omega-3s are eliminated. Industrial meat raised on seeds rather than leaves, have fewer omega-3s and more omega-6s than preindustrial meat used to have.

Official dietary advice since the 1970s has promoted the consumption of polyunsaturated vegetable oils, most of which are high in omega-6s (corn and soy especially). Thus, without realizing what we were doing, we significantly altered the ratio of these two essential fats in our diets and bodies, with the result that the ratio of omega-6 to omega-3 in the typical American today stands at more than 10 to 1; before the widespread introduction of seed oils at the turn of the last century, it was closer to 1 to 1.

Responding to an alarming increase in chronic diseases linked to diet — including heart disease, cancer and diabetes — a Senate Select Committee on Nutrition, headed by George McGovern, held hearings on the problem and prepared what by all rights should have been an uncontroversial document called "Dietary Goals for the United States."

The committee learned that while rates of coronary heart disease had soared in America since World War II, other cultures consuming traditional diets based largely on plants had strikingly low rates of chronic disease. Epidemiologists also had observed that in America during the war years, when meat and dairy products were strictly rationed, the rate of heart disease temporarily plummeted.

The Year of Eating Oat Bran — also known as 1988 — served as a kind of coming-out party for the food scientists, who succeeded in getting the ingredient into nearly every processed food sold in America. Oat bran's moment on the dietary stage didn't last long, but the pattern had been established, and every few years since then, a new oat bran has taken its turn under the marketing lights. (Here comes omega-3!)

Consider what happened immediately after the 1977 "Dietary Goals" — McGovern's masterpiece of politico-nutritionist compromise. In the wake of the panel's recommendation that we cut down on saturated fat, a recommendation seconded by the 1982 National Academy report on cancer, Americans did indeed change their diets, endeavoring for a quarter-century to do what they had been told. Well, kind of. The industrial food supply was promptly reformulated to reflect the official advice, giving us low-fat pork, low-fat Snackwell's and all the low-fat pasta and high-fructose (yet low-fat!) corn syrup we could consume, which turned out to be quite a lot.

Oddly, America got really fat on its new low-fat diet — indeed, many date the current obesity and diabetes epidemic to the late 1970s, when Americans began binging on carbohydrates, ostensibly as a way to avoid the evils of fat. It was easy for the take-home message of the 1977 and 1982 dietary guidelines to be simplified as follows: eat more low-fat foods. And that is what we did.

BUDGETING TIME AND MONEY

A Simple Start

You can make healthy choices as a family, one small step at a time. Even small changes in your routine can help save money. And getting started doesn't take much time.

Make a shopping list. Keep a shopping list in place easy to see so you can add to it any time. Checking your list as you shop can help you stick to your budget. Children can help write or draw items on the list, or check things off while shopping.

Look for generic or store brands. These usually cost less than name brands and taste just as good!

Start the day with a healthy breakfast. A healthy breakfast gives the whole family energy to stay focused all day. It can also be the most affordable meal of the day, whether you make it at home or participate in a public school breakfast program. You can get creative with breakfast, too — try a healthy breakfast burrito with beans, salsa, low-fat cheese, and a whole wheat tortilla.

Thinking Ahead

Whether you are shopping at a large supermarket, a farmers market, or a local grocery store, simple steps can help you save money. Spend just a few minutes planning ahead and you can save a lot of time and money in the long run!

Planning ahead gets easier over time. The whole family can help make choices that fit into your routines.

Buy fruits and vegetables in season. Although most fruits and vegetables are available throughout the year, keep in mind some cost less when they are in season. Farmers markets offer seasonal produce, and many accept SNAP cards or WIC vouchers. To find out what's in season, search for "seasonal produce" online, or ask someone working in your local market.

Buy in bulk. You may save money by buying in bulk (if you will use large quantities) or stocking up on sale items. Grab a family member or a friend or 2 and buy in bulk with them. Use the day to meal prep together. You'll find it won't only be cheaper doing it together, but it's a great way to bond with family members or friends about the meals for the week ahead.

Be in the know. Find out when stores publish weekly flyers or announce sale items. Ask a store manager or clerk about current or upcoming sales. Are you single and use the excuse that you buy too much and it goes to waste? Ask your produce department in the market if they offer to cut the produce in half and sell it for half the price. This is becoming very common in most cities and states.

In the Long Term

There are even more steps your family can take to make healthy choices on a budget over time. You can make healthy choices as a family, one small step at a time. Even small changes in your routine can help save money. And getting started doesn't take much time.

Create a weekly menu. As you get used to planning ahead, preparing weekly menus can help you save money and make food last longer. Planning ahead for your meals of the week helps you stay on track. When you buy the ingredients, make sure you have enough for the week.

Plant a garden. Growing your own food can be a great way to have fun as a family and save money. Plant things like tomatoes, peppers, and herbs outdoors or in pots at home, or look for community gardens in your area. Gardening helps children learn where food comes from — they will also be excited to try the healthy foods that they helped grow. Don't have a garden? Look for a community garden or pay it forward by donating your time to local charities or schools that help build gardens and organic awareness.

Stay healthy on weekends and during the summer. You may find summer breakfast programs, weekend services or community meals in your neighborhood. You may also find free summer activity programs or events, such as playground playtime, where your child can get healthy snacks, too.

Stretch Your Dollar

These tips can help you make healthy hearty meals that fit your budget.

- **Choose low-cost resources of protein.** Dried beans, peas, and lentils; canned fish; eggs; and peanut butter are healthy, inexpensive sources of protein.

- **Buy frozen or canned fruits and vegetables.** In addition to fresh produce, try to pick canned food that is labeled "in its own juice," "no added sugar," or "low sodium." If these aren't available, drain and rinse other types before eating. Frozen vegetables are picked and frozen when the food is most fresh and are a great alternative when your favorites aren't in season; they're also useful if you're in a time crunch.

- **Swap foods and coupons with friends.** You may have many cans or boxes of food, or extra coupons. Ask friends if they have different extra items or coupons to exchange. Swapping can help you add variety to your meals — and save money, too!

- **Try powdered milk.** Its long shelf life makes it an easy, affordable option. You can you use it instead of regular milk in just about any recipe, from creamed vegetable soups to rich fruit smoothies.

Save For Later

Leftovers can be made into delicious and healthy meals. At home, save time and money by making more servings than you need, then saving the rest.

- **Refrigerate or freeze leftovers quickly.** If you plan to eat leftovers within a day or so, refrigerate them. If you plan to eat them later than that, freeze leftovers in reusable containers.
- **Thaw foods safely.** Leaving foods to thaw on the counter can make them unsafe to eat. Thaw foods safely in the refrigerator, in cold water, or in the microwave.
- **Divide portion sizes.** Separate leftovers into single serving sizes for easy preparation.
- **Mark and date food.** To keep track of when you put the foods in the freezer or refrigerator, mark the containers with the date and what's inside.

CLIENT STORY: WALKER

I had been a trainer for about 4 years when I got a call one morning from a man named Walker. Walker was a soft-spoken man with a hint of a drawl. He found my ad months before but something in him decided it was time to give me a call. Walker was 34 years old, but according to his recent physical, his doctor measured his age to be over the age of 60. He stands 5'11" and weighs 340 pounds.

Walker was an engineer, lived alone, and had been single for the last few years. He was originally from a small Baptist town in Tennessee. He was the youngest of 4 kids and the only one who had ever moved away from home. His parents had been married for over 40 years. His two brothers and sister were married, and between the 3 of them had 7 kids. Walker loved to open up about his family, but when it came to his own personal life he was vague.

When Walker came in the following day for a consultation one of the first things I noticed was how sad his eyes were and how much pain he seemed to be in — not just physically, but emotionally as well. Every move he made was around his own body image. He was constantly tugging out his shirt, crossing his arms and trying to ignore the fact he was sweating heavily from the half of block walk he made and his nerves.

Walker began to train with me consistently twice a week. When it came time for his first 6-week evaluation, I noticed significant change and advancement with balance, technique and his knowledge about certain body parts and equipment. His shoulders were no longer hunched, his weight no longer shifted to his right side, and now both feet were rooted in the ground. I was proud of his hard work and dedication to the hours we had worked together. The big issue and elephant in the room was that in 6 weeks he had only lost 5 pounds. No question he worked hard with the 4% (one hour) of his day when we trained — but it was what he was doing, or not doing, the rest of the 23 hours that irked me.

When we sat down to discuss the assessment Walker swore he was eating nothing but lean meat, complex carbs and a ton of vegetables. He acted like the perfect student reciting what I had been telling him to eat and the importance of water. From his physical, I knew Walker did not have a thyroid issue and levels according to his blood work came back normal.

This is why I knew he was lying and it was impossible that at his weight he was not losing at least 3 pounds a week. I believe fundamentals to weight loss start with exerting more calories than you take in. This is why it did not add up and this was not my first rodeo with excuses and people who make them.

He had every excuse in the book and was "fathomed" and blamed it on his slow metabolism he knew ran in his family. I liked Walker, knew he wasn't being honest with himself or me, but liked him enough to continue working with him for the next 6 weeks that ended the same as the weeks before. He continued to tell me how well he was eating, how he was waking up early to do cardio and how proud of himself he was. I continued to try to get him to open up about his weight gain history and his triggers.

Walker was in shock when, at the next 6-week evaluation, I fired him as a client. I kindly explained that without him being open and honest, there was nothing more I could do to help him succeed. He tried to fight me saying I was being abusive and I was ridiculous for not continuing to work with him because he wasn't living up to my "unrealistic standards." His voice was the only one raised and as many hurtful words he projected my way, I was silently relieved he did have some fight in him and passion. I wished him the best and reminded him that losing weight was a mental, physical and spiritual journey. I couldn't tell if he heard what I said over all his profanity until a month and a half later.

May 16th was a Wednesday that year. I had just finished up with my 5th client of the day and was packing up to meet my boyfriend at the time for dinner. Like a movie, I heard a familiar voice asking me if I thought "I could run him off that easy." The minute I saw him I ran to hug him. I had no idea if my tough love tactic would work with him but I knew he needed something and someone to make him accountable for his actions if he wanted to grow.

He explained to me after he left me that day he went to McDonald's and ordered 4 Big Macs, 2 Quarter Pounders and supersized the fries and chocolate milkshake. This was not an unusual order for him, but it was the first time he began to think about what he was eating, how much and why he hid in his car while he was eating. He said in that moment is when he had his breakthrough and in turn I had mine as well; I had the inspiration for my company Ferrigno FIT.

There was nothing soft-spoken about Walker when he told me he was gay, and I was the first person he had come out to. When he noticed I didn't run, gasp, drop my jaw and call him a homo (his biggest fear about coming out) he continued to explain. He told me he would eat to suppress his sexuality. Because his family is very religious, he believed they would "disown him" if they ever found out; he ate so no one would be interested in him sexually.

This is when it all came together. It explained why he was so hesitant to open up, why he moved away from his hometown, and why he allowed himself to carry an extra 125 pounds on his 5'11" frame. It was his shame, in return for his secret, that he meant to "keep unknown and unseen by others." But what he realized in the McDonald's parking lot was that he wasn't fooling anyone by being 360 pounds. All his dishonesty did was leave him alone and keep him in the abusive relationship he had with food. He realized he was hiding nothing by being as big as he was. I made a deal with him that we would continue to train but he would have to do the emotional and spiritual work on himself as well. He agreed to begin therapy and he agreed that when he was ready he would come out to his family.

AA has an expression that "you're only as sick as your secrets," and I believe it's true with any addiction. With food I believe "You're only as FIT as your secrets." You're not 340 pounds because you like to eat, and you're not necessarily an alcoholic because you like to drink. We mask and divert our secrets and truth with substances. We suppress and self-sabotage to mask what is going on inside, things we don't want to face or don't know where to start with facing them.

After countless hours of therapy and 28 pounds lighter, Walker stayed true to his word. He flew home to Tennessee to come out to his family. No one disowned him, called him derogatory words, or threw up at his truth. If anything, most confirmed they knew or had a suspicion since he was a kid. His parents admitted they were not thrilled at the idea, but told him they didn't love him any less and they wanted him to live a long and healthy life as God intended him to.

That same year Walker lost another 94 pounds — a 122-pound total, bringing him from 340 to a muscular 218 pounds. Walker now runs, does Mud runs, works out with his partner 5x a week, and has continued to keep the weight off. Coming out and no longer keeping his truth a secret was the heavy weight. Once that was lifted relearning how to have a relationship with food came easy. Throughout that year working with Walker gave me the strength to begin to look at my journey and why I myself had struggled for so long with weight issues.

EXCUSE #9:
MY PAST WILL ALWAYS HAUNT ME AND I'LL ALWAYS BE THIS WAY – IT'S JUST WHO I AM

This excuse can actually be true, *if* you allow it: if you are an adult, you're in charge of your own happiness. If you are overweight today, that isn't your parent's fault. You control what you eat at this stage of your life. You're in control of your feelings and how you deal with them. You picked up this book for a reason. It is time to accept your past is what it is, and let go of what was.

Every day is another opportunity to reset. Your future is in your own hands.

NATURE VS. NURTURE

Many people blame their genetics for excess weight gain and therefore, make very little effort to exercise. The "it's in my genetics" argument is an excuse to do nothing or not exercise at all. While genetics may play a role, environmental factors can override obesity. Being predisposed to weight gain is not a necessary cause of obesity, but more of an underlying problem. The problem is, many people who think they can't lose weight because of their genetics, tend to overeat. Psychologists call this a self-fulfilling prophecy. It is possible to lose weight, regardless of your genetics.

I realize losing weight can be an uphill battle, but the very fact that you are reading this book is already a step in the right direction. Learn about the foods making us fat, such as Genetically Modified Foods (GMOs) that might be "stronger" and "better" but are also making us fat. We need to go back to a simpler time when it comes to our food. Ask yourself, "Would your great-grandmother serve this food on her table?"

Eating a diet free of GMOs or scientific advances is the only way to go. We need to go back to nature and eat only fresh fruits, vegetables, plants or meats that are *not* genetically modified. Our body cannot process GMOs, and eliminating them from our diet is the best solution. You would think it would be easy to spot GMO foods, such as pre-packaged foods, but even though it has "all-natural" or "organic" on the label does not mean that you should eat it. Look for foods that are labeled "non-GMO" and focus on organically-grown produce. Nurturing your body with non-GMO foods is a great place to start.

When it comes to losing weight, going back to nature instead of eating GMO foods is an excellent way to nurture your health and lose weight in the process. Not all scientific advances in technology are good for our body — in fact, they need to stay out of our food supply. Nurture your body with non-GMO, healthy, natural food, the way nature intended.

THE POWER OF LETTING GO

Being heavy is a burden that no one should have to endure or share. It might mean eating something to numb your emotions and avoid crying, or simply choosing McDonald's for dinner because you have forgotten how to listen to your body. I am a huge supporter of crying. I believe it melts the ice around your heart. Crying gives us a natural cleanse, both mentally and physically. It's especially important to cry if you feel like crying when you are stressed. Tears produced by stress help the body get rid of cortisol — the stress hormone we talk about extensively throughout the book. Crying through your feelings instead of masking them with food or alcohol, according to a 2008 study from the University of South Florida, is the best self-soothing technique and elevates mood better than any antidepressant.

Ask your hypothalamus — it is the major control gland of your endocrine system that lets you know how much fat to store and how hungry you are. It is driven by our need to survive. For some of you, it means eating what your family eats, letting your weight push people away and being fat to being overweight to validate a belief that you are not good enough. If you listen to your body, you will find your own built-in safety mechanisms hidden in the deep reserves of your body fat.

However, being overweight or fat is not a safe option for anyone. Life is too short and you should feel free in your body and be the most powerful person you can be. You have too many gifts and things to offer to the world to waste your time being overweight. Getting back to your best or when you were your slimmest is a journey and it may take some time unravel the years of self-abuse. It will take some work and lifestyle changes but trust me. Eventually, you will look forward to that leafy green salad.

You will learn how to exercise the right way, move your body, and not because you are trying to control it, but because it makes you feel good. You *will* learn to love yourself and accept yourself for who you are right now, at this very moment, fat and all. Accepting yourself how you are right now is the only way to get lean. That may sound counter-intuitive, but your happiness comes from within, not the outside of you.

Losing weight can be a joyous journey. Sometimes we may look in the mirror and get frustrated or depressed because the physical changes are not coming fast enough. You might think, "I have been so dedicated, and nothing is happening." However, that is simply not true.

When you commit to being healthy and losing weight, you commit to living by a new wisdom and a new way of living. You are no longer a victim of mirrors or the weight scale. You believe in yourself with every cell in your body, even if it has not manifested yet, it will. Remind yourself of that daily. You can let go of your body fat and the pain of it every single moment. When you focus on being healthy right now, you release the burden of worrying about how much weight you will lose in the future.

Remind yourself gently and be kind to yourself. You are free to make the choice to let go of any weight you are holding on to. It really is that easy.

REDEFINING YOU

C.S. Lewis was quoted as saying, "You are never too old to set another goal or dream a new dream." What does that mean? It means every time we make a major change in our life — such as moving to a new city, leaving a relationship or job and even losing a loved one — we must take control of who we will become or risk never reaching our potential. Change means reinvention. Most of us have had to reinvent ourselves several times in our lifetime. However, what we should be doing is "choosing to reinvent ourselves."

Forging a new path deliberately with forethought, prudence and anticipation is exciting. Instead of waiting for our future to find us, waiting in vain and feeling lost or confused, we sometimes end up in a situation we didn't want or imagine. We might have trouble moving forward partly because we have no idea what we want to move forward to, thinking about our past and realizing it is not what we want for our future.

Here are some steps to consider in order to redefine YOU and take control of your future:

Step 1: Create A Vision Of What You Want To Look Like
Take a moment and sit quietly, close your eyes and imagine the physique you would like to have. Imagine what it will feel like to wear the clothes you want and

have the energy to do anything you want. Silently voice your appreciation for your body and health. With gratitude and compassion, imagine yourself walking away from an unhealthy you to a healthy, slim you.

Step 2: Make A Specific Plan

Write out what you are willing to do. Keep a journal to record your meals and make note of how you are feeling before and after a meal. Keep your journal with you and make the changes that you need to do. For example, eat more vegetables at meal times. Exercise daily.

Step 3: Use Visual Reminders

Whether it is post-its or images from a magazine of what you want to look like, put them someplace where you will see those images every single day. The image or note can be anything that reminds you of what you are moving toward.

Step 4: Break It Up Into Workable Tasks

What do you need to change in your current lifestyle so you can be healthier? Be specific. For example, if you have been skipping breakfast, create a list of meals for breakfast you will eat. Are you missing your workouts? Schedule them — make an appointment with yourself. Then do it — and commit to it one day at a time.

Step 5: Every Day, Revisit Your New Vision Of YOU

Every morning or every evening, take a moment to close your eyes and see yourself as a slimmer version of you — a healthy you. Reconnect with why you are moving toward redefining you.

The road to redefining you is not always smooth or easy. You may encounter difficulties, resistance to working out, making the necessary changes to a healthier lifestyle. You may not want to let go of old habits or junk food, even though we know they are not good for you. You might still struggle with limiting beliefs about yourself or don't want to try new things — like kale, ha! However, there is one way to keep your compass pointing towards the new you, even in the midst of any struggles or resistance you may encounter along the way.

Every time you find yourself slipping into old, bad habits, ask yourself, "What can I do right now to keep moving forward?"

Don't beat yourself up or keep wondering why you couldn't resist those cinnamon buns in the mall. No matter what you are feeling at that moment — lazy, exhausted, disappointed or self-critical — do something to maintain your momentum, no matter how small. Drink some water, put your gym shoes on and go for a walk. True courage is not about feeling fearful — it is about feeling those fears and acting on them anyway. Be courageous instead of letting your fear choose the future of you. You are worth it and deserve it.

FORGIVING SOMEONE

Whether it is a holiday or special occasion, you might be the type of person who honors those you love with gifts, cards, or other special items; however, you need to honor the most important relationship there is: the one you have with your own body. Love your body unconditionally as you create positive and permanent results with your physique. When I say, "forgiving someone," I am talking about forgiving yourself. That might sound simple, but if you are like most of my clients on their weight loss journey, you can be relentless when it comes to criticizing yourself, specifically your body.

When you let go of the shame and guilt about how you look or what you might have done to your body over the years, you enter a world of positivity and love that will help you create the healthy body that you so desperately want and deserve. When you forgive yourself, you can release negative judgments and you are less likely to act on those negative feelings. It becomes second nature to take better care of your body. When you love yourself unconditionally and forgive yourself more easily, you are more likely to eat healthier foods, treat yourself to a workout, and be more compassionate to YOU.

On the other hand, when you are feeling sad, depressed, or angry towards yourself, you are more likely to turn to junk for comfort or even to punish yourself. Those negative feelings can get out of control, quickly turning you into a victim instead of being in charge. When you develop the habit of forgiving yourself, you will notice subtle changes in your health. You no longer rely on junk food for comfort. When you love yourself, you are less likely to skip that body sculpting class at the gym or your personal training session.

Forgiving yourself takes persistence and patience. Be open to the healing power of forgiving yourself. Love yourself and bring peace to your heart and mind. Remember, happiness comes from within. Here are some strategies to consider:

Be Willing To Release Self-Hatred Of Your Body — Forgiving yourself is about being willing to release shame, self-hatred, and guilt about your body. Set an intention to do this today. Simply say, "I forgive myself." Love yourself fully and treat yourself with kindness. Stop berating yourself and stop the cycle of emotional eating. When you forgive yourself, you take charge of your health and your life.

Focus Your Attention On Your Heart — It is easy to fall back into old patterns of unhealthy eating or not exercising. Should this happen to you, do not dwell on negative feelings or thoughts and remind yourself that you can stop right now. Take a deep breath and turn your attention towards your heart. Think about a happy memory or someone you love. It can help you feel calm right away and forgive yourself.

Enjoy Quiet — Take some time each day to connect with your breath. If you are familiar with yoga or practice yoga on a daily basis, one of the first things you learn to do is to connect with your breath in the quiet. It teaches you to accept yourself with all of your limitations and connect with the loving energy of your heart. Notice and watch the sensations you feel when you simply focus on your breath without any judgment. Know that you are loved by the pure energy within you.

When you practice the above steps on a regular basis, you will begin to create a lightness of spirit that is within you. Have faith and be patient. Over time, you will notice the love you give to yourself on the inside will reflect in the way that you take care of your body. You can do it with confidence and love.

YOUR MAINTENANCE PROGRAM

The same strategies and methods that help you lose weight will not necessarily help you keep the weight off. In other words, once you have achieved your goals, you may need to switch gears in order to maintain your weight loss. As you go through the weight loss process, you learned different behaviors and skill sets such as eliminating sugar from your diet, not skipping meals and eating healthy snacks. However, while these practices are important, they do not have much to do with *maintaining* your weight loss.

Following a consistent exercise program, eating high-quality, low-fat sources of protein, and reminding yourself why you want to maintain a healthy weight will help you maintain it. It can be similar to love and marriage. In other words, what gets you to the altar is quite different than what keeps you married for the long haul. If you do not recognize the transition and adapt with different strategies, you can get into trouble in more ways than one. Losing weight is the easy part; maintaining it is another story.

Yes, it still comes down to eliminating junk food or sugar, getting regular exercise, etc. — but the practices that help you achieve those are different. You must switch your mindset to a more permanent way of living so you can keep the weight off for good. People want to concentrate on losing weight but the hard part is keeping it off. You need to create the right kind of strategies that work for you and reinforce both a healthy diet and exercise. Successful maintenance of weight loss requires changing your mindset.

If you want to lose weight, stay healthy, and keep it off, you need to change the way you eat. The first three letters in the word "diet" spell "die," implying a beginning and an end that sets you up for failure. Keeping the weight off and being healthy must become a lifelong habit. You have to change your relationship to food for the rest of your life. It takes planning and knowing what and when you are going to eat. There is nothing worse than being starved and on fast-food row. You must plan your meals just like you plan what you are going to wear the next day at work or scheduling your child's week ahead. You might have to pack your own lunch and not skip meals.

GIVING BACK

There is nothing better than giving back to those around you and the ones you love. Giving back what you have learned from your experience losing weight is invaluable to all that know you. Seeing how far you can go and experiencing that balance that is so important to all of us is priceless. When you share your knowledge and give back to those around you, camaraderie is built and it becomes more of a team effort instead of an individual effort. Everyone wins.

CLIENT STORY: CHRISTINA

Christina was 27 years old when she came to one of my fitness workshops I was hosting at the time. At 5'6" tall and an Italian American, Christina was big-boned and had always been a little overweight, no matter how athletic she was at the time. When she started college, her hours became longer and her classes became tougher. She worked out less often, but continued to eat and drink what she wanted without thinking about it. Sometimes, she would only eat one big meal a day, skip breakfast, and then drink at night. She tried to get into the gym, but since her nutrition was awful, she was always too tired.

Like most of us, she was "guilted" into finishing everything on her plate growing up. If she didn't, she couldn't leave the table without permission. She overate a lot and it wasn't healthy food. At 14, she started trying to lose weight by fad-dieting. She would try starving herself, eat the same frozen meals every day or eat only eat veggies, to name a few; but nothing worked. After fad dieting, her body craved junk food at such a heavy rate, Christina not only went back to her original weight, she gained 15 pounds more. The cycle kept going like this for years.

Sill heavy and searching for happiness, Christina graduated college and decided to move across the country from Michigan to California. She landed a corporate job, thinking she found the answer to her dreams. Instead, she felt alone and was sedentary all day and gained even more weight.

Between the office parties and team lunches that included unlimited amounts of fried foods, pizza, cookies, cakes, etc., trying to bond and fit in was literally killing her, and she was still unhappy with the person she had become. She was no longer an athlete, her clothes were too small, and her confidence disappeared. This is when she knew something needed to change... *she* needed to change.

Christina and I started together a month after she came to my workshop. I began to teach her about the importance of eating small meals throughout the day and what to look for on the labels. We talked, in length, about how important it is, at any size, to love yourself first. No matter if she moved to the moon, she was still going to hold on to the same eating patterns and mentality that were formed when she was young, if she didn't reset the pattern and identify the triggers. I was able to get a few pounds off that way.

Christina took to her *Reset Plan* really well and she got down to 138 pounds. Her success came from focusing on self-happiness and positivity with life. She concentrated on checking in with what made her happy inside, rather than repressing her emotions with food. She was happy with the weight loss but more than anything I watched her become happy and confident with herself.

She started to pay it forward in her community by volunteering at the local Boys And Girls Club, which included community functions such as 5K walks and runs. By staying busy and joining other groups that were positive and healthy, it helped her not obsess over food or how fast or slow the weight was coming off.

I saw Christina a year later and she looked better than ever. She admitted that after breaking up with a boyfriend, she went back to some old patterns and gained back 9 pounds of her old weight. I see that happen a lot after a huge weight loss and that is really normal. The coolest part about catching up with her was that no matter what weight, she was happy. She ate healthy and kept those 9 pounds as her goal weight, but not as an obsession.

EXCUSE #10:
I CAN EAT ANYTHING I WANT
BECAUSE I PLAN TO WORK OUT LATER

Sometimes when people are exercising more than they used to, or even feeling pretty good about how they are looking, they start to think, "I can eat this cake [or pizza or candy] because I am going to work out later." This chapter discusses why life is not usually that simple, life gets hectic and we aren't always in control with what our day-to-day might bring. If you want to stay on track it is *so* important you eat for the work you did, not what you're going to do.

It's not that people can't treat themselves, but they need to make sure they have earned or budgeted for those extra calories if they are trying to stay in a weight loss or maintenance phase. This chapter explores maintenance. The plan this week asks readers to perform the fitness assessment exercises again and compare the results with previous performance, offers specific guidance and detailed options for increasing cardio workouts and strength training exercises, goals for daily water consumption, and includes the weekly household project, and journaling topics.

EATING ACCORDING TO *YOUR* GOALS

Whatever your specific fitness goals are, exercising alone is not enough. You must eat according to your fitness goals. Healthy eating is not just about losing weight. It is important for good health, more energy, and to function at optimum levels throughout the day. While a specific goal may require you to eat in a slightly different way, there are some specific guidelines you need to follow regardless of your fitness goal. Here are some healthy guidelines to follow that will help support all of your hard work at the gym:

Track Your Diet — Just because your best friend lost weight eating nothing but cabbage soup, it does not mean this is going to work for you or that she will even keep the weight off long term. There is no one diet that works for everyone. There is not one specific *Reset Plan* that will work for every person. Follow *The Reset Plan* guidelines your way.

No matter what religious or spiritual truth you believe or take in as fact, at each and every different stage in your life, though the words remain the same for hundreds or thousands of years, you will internalize it differently than you did a day, a month, or years ago. No matter with whom you discuss religion or spirituality, it will always have a different meaning to everyone, though the words remain the same, and have since they were written. I feel the same about *The Reset Plan*. I hope you follow and take in the blueprint, but enjoy the journey as your own. Track your meals and make changes based on what works for you. It will also help you figure out what doesn't work for you.

Think WHOLE Foods — Cut out the processed foods and create meals around whole foods. If a food item has more than five ingredients and an expiration date, you do not want to eat it. Eliminate the foods that have a hundred different ingredients that you probably can't pronounce. Buy locally and go to farmers markets on the weekend for fresh produce.

Do NOT Rely On Labels — Even if it is gluten-free or low in fat, it doesn't mean the food is healthy. Labels are designed to sell you a product. Just because something says it is healthy, it does not mean it is. Build meals around whole, natural foods. If you find wheat or gluten sets off allergic reactions, irritable bowel syndrome or other symptoms, then you may find that you feel better without eating wheat. If you have been diagnosed with celiac disease, then the gluten-free way of life is for you — and, of course, you should always follow your doctor's recommendations.

Start With The Basics — And keep it simple. Do not worry about always having a variety. Choose a few healthy food items and build a meal plan around them. Find recipes that incorporate these foods with all natural spices and herbs. If you have found a meal that works for you, don't worry about changing it up right away. Preparing a healthy meal well will help you get into a rhythm for prepping meals, and that will make it easier to stick with your healthy eating plan.

Plan, Plan, Plan — Preparation is important. If you are not prepared, you can make an excuse for deviating from your meal plan. The easiest way to plan ahead is to cook meals that will give you plenty of leftovers for the week.

Learn To Use A Crockpot — Crockpots allow you to create large quantities of food for the week with very easy preparation. For example, add chicken, vegetables, and tomato sauce to the crockpot in the morning and come home to a delicious home-cooked meal without any fuss. (See recipes in The *Reset Plan Workbook*.)

Plan For Travel — Are you going to stay on your eating plan or throw it out the window? A great way to prepare for trips or meals out with friends is to choose restaurants that offer healthy options. The more you are prepared for these situations, the more you will be able to stick with your healthy eating plan. If you do cheat, get right back on your eating plan the very next meal.

Follow The 80/20 Rule — Do not expect to eat perfectly every day at every single meal. Expecting to be perfect all the time can set you up for failure and feeling guilty. Allow yourself to indulge in a special treat once in a while — once a week is fine. Some people do well with one "maintenance" meal per week, while others do better with a little treat each day. Find out what works for you. Love yourself, trust your support network, and trust your *Reset Plan*.

Eat When You Are Hungry — Now, this doesn't mean to skip breakfast if you wake up and are not hungry — otherwise, you might binge later, feeling starved. Listen to your body. On the days you do not exercise, you might not be as hungry. Eat based on the amount of activity you do each day.

Drink Water — Staying hydrated is one of the most important things you can do. Many times, we feel hungry, when in reality we are actually thirsty. Do not wait until you are thirsty. A well-hydrated body means a well-functioning metabolism. Drinking enough water each day can prevent you from eating extra calories and help your body burn calories.

Eat Good Fats — Fat does not make you fat. Eating good fats from avocados and nuts, for example, can actually help you lose weight. Fat will keep you full longer and are very good for your health. Other good choices are coconut, fatty fish like salmon, and extra-virgin olive oil.

Make sure you understand why you are eating the healthy foods you choose. Do not just follow an eating plan blindly because your best friend says it's healthy. Experiment with different whole foods and determine which ones you like the best and help yield results from all of your hard work in the gym. Track what you are doing and make changes as you progress. If you don't track what you are doing, then it will be more difficult to figure out what you should continue to do and what you should change.

USING RULES AND PLANS

First and foremost, having a weight loss goal can make the difference between failure and enjoying success. Using rules and plans can help you stay focused and motivated. They can provide a plan for positive changes you learn to eat in a healthier manner. Many weight loss goals are quite helpful, while others can be overly strict and undermine your efforts to lose weight. Use rules and plans that work for you, not against you.

While you may have a specific weight loss goal, you need to know and understand how to achieve it. For example, a good plan is to aim for more fruits and vegetables each day and drink plenty of water each day. Focus on changing behaviors and habits that are necessary for losing weight. Setting smart goals each day that are specific will help you stay on track and are measureable. For example, eating healthier meals is not easily measured but knowing how many calories you are consuming each day is.

If your work schedule does not allow you to spend an hour in the gym each day, then you may have to find ways to squeeze exercise in throughout the day. You can plan on going to the gym on the weekends. You have to be realistic and figure out what is going to work for you to be successful. If your goals, and how you are going to reach them, are unrealistic, you will feel disappointed when you don't reach them. You may be tempted to give up altogether.

Fitness goals are best achieved if you keep a record of your progress. Keep a journal, and let it be your friend. It is an excellent way to keep track of and evaluate your progress each day. It can help you shift your thinking from simply being "on a diet" to making lifestyle changes that work for you. You can break down a long-term goal into a series of short-term or smaller goals. For example, if your goal is to lose 15 pounds, perhaps you can break it down into 5 pounds each month.

Anyone and everyone who has ever made the effort to make changes experience setbacks. It is part of making changes in your life, especially when it comes to losing weight. You have to expect them, and develop a plan for dealing with any setbacks. For example, if you have a family reunion coming up or it's the holidays, come up with strategies to help you stay on course. I can help you do this.

You have to be willing to change your goals as you make progress. Reassess and adjust your fitness goals as needed. If you are able to achieve success with each goal you set, you might be ready to take on bigger challenges. In fact, you might have to adjust your goals to better fit your new, healthy lifestyle.

DID YOU SIGN UP FOR AN EVENT YET?

Signing up for a 10K walk or a local triathlon will automatically give you a specific goal and challenge that can ignite a fire in you to succeed. Of course, you should register for a competition or event that is within reason of your current abilities and fitness level. If you sign up for an event that is way out of your league, you could leave feeling unmotivated and wanting to give up. Health maintenance organizations, health insurance carriers, and medical centers are good places to contact to find local event and walking groups, for example.

Check your local fitness or running shoe stores for publications and brochures that list running and walking clubs as well as fitness events. Some stores have their own walking and running clubs that meet regularly to walk or run together. This is a great way to get involved in your community, meet people and make registering for a fitness event more of a reality. Health clubs often sponsor many fitness events, running groups, walking events, and, in some areas, racquetball competitions. You might also look for charity walking events and invite your family and friends to participate with you. By participating in an event with a family member or friend, it can make it less intimidating and a fun way to spend time together. Again — have you signed up for an event yet? Do it now.

EXERCISE AND APPETITE SUPPRESSION

New studies show that when you perform a vigorous workout on a treadmill, it affects two key appetite hormones, ghrelin and peptide YY, while 90 minutes of weight lifting affects the level of ghrelin hormone only. In other words, aerobic exercise is better at suppressing appetite than weight lifting alone, and provides effective ways to use exercise for controlling weight. (American Journal of Physiology-Regulatory, Integrative and Comparative Physiology, published by The American Physiological Society)

There are several hormones that help regulate appetite, however ghrelin is the only hormone to stimulate appetite. Peptide YY suppresses appetite. The studies show that an aerobic session caused ghrelin levels to drop and peptide YY levels to increase, indicating the hormones suppress appetite. However, weight training produces a mixed result. Ghrelin levels drop causing appetite suppression, but peptide YY levels do not change significantly. Both aerobic and weight training suppress hunger, but aerobic exercise produces a greater suppression of appetite or hunger.

Ghrelin comes in two forms: acylated (or active ghrelin) and non-acylated. Active ghrelin can cross the blood-brain barrier and reach the appetite center in the brain. The studies suggest future research needs to concentrate on active ghrelin. And while the studies show exercise suppresses appetite hormones, the next step should be to establish whether this change actually causes the suppression of eating. Regardless of the studies, since you have been exercising regularly and eating healthier, no doubt, you have noticed a difference in your appetite in a good way. You probably have noticed you are not very hungry after a hard workout, all the more reason to keep on keeping on with your health and fitness goals.

HOUSEHOLD PROJECTS; LESSONS LEARNED

There is a lot of misinformation out there about weight loss and diet. You can find an endless supply of content geared towards selling you a particular diet or product which is often exaggerated when it comes to their effectiveness for weight loss. Based on my personal experience, there are several common missing factors you must understand in order to have successful weight loss.

First and foremost, you have to eat in order to lose weight. In fact, you can eat too little food and not see results. Your body uses food as fuel to build muscle and burn body fat. If you don't eat enough food, your body cannot work properly and it will hold on to fat. The biggest mistake I see "beginner dieters" make is cut their caloric-intake way too low. Think of muscle as your body's furnace that burns calories all the time, even when you are not exercising — that is the benefit of strength training. Your body continues to burn calories hours after your workout.

Keep doing your cardiovascular and weight training workout as well as eating healthy and you will lose fat. Your body decides where it will come off first. Just because you want to lose fat in your belly, it doesn't matter how many abdominal crunches you do, you will not lose belly fat any faster. Building muscle through weight training will give you a well-toned body when you do lose body fat.

Eating all low-fat foods is not necessary — in other words, fat does not make you fat. Healthy fats are always good to incorporate into your eating plan: avocados, olive oil, nuts, seeds, and other fatty foods like salmon are all good choices. Of course, enjoy all good things in moderation. The same goes for carbohydrates. Healthy carbohydrates like fresh fruits, vegetables, beans and nuts are vitally important for any balanced diet. What makes you fat is consuming too many calories overall that are not nutrient-dense.

Beware of foods labeled "healthy" or "diet" or any health claims because they usually are covering up the negative things about that particular food. If the food is labeled "low-fat," then it is probably full of artificial flavorings, preservatives, and chemicals and high in carbohydrates. In other words, you are better off eating less of the real thing than something labeled "light" or "low-fat." Read the ingredient list and pay attention to any health claims. Better yet, eat whole foods that do not come in a package.

Be careful when going out to restaurants, as portions are way out of control, even for salads. Many entrées in restaurants have over 2,000 calories with their enormous portions. Ask for a take-out container when you order your entrée and place half of it in the box when it arrives. Most entrées serve up enough portions for two to three meals.

Do not base your day on what the scale says. It really is not an accurate measurement of your health or weight loss efforts. Weight fluctuates from day to day and depending on the food you ate, water retention, or other physiological processes; it is simply impossible to gain or lose fat or weight of two pounds per day. These fluctuations are quite normal and should not stress you out. Measure your progress by how you look and how your clothes are fitting and take the time to appreciate your improved fitness and cardiovascular level.

Make sure you eat a healthy meal before and after your workout. A small snack before your workout will give you that extra energy that can help push you during your workout. After your workout, enjoy a protein snack that will help your body repair muscle and recover. You do not build muscle or lose body fat in the gym; it happens later as you recover from your workout. Make sure you give your body the right fuel so you see results from all of your hard workouts.

Exercise with intensity — it is okay to sweat. Get your heart rate up while doing cardiovascular exercise. Challenge yourself by adding heavier weights when it's warranted — this goes for women, too. Women do not have enough testosterone to get large muscles. Overall, listen to your body, and when you feel hungry, think of it as a sign to fuel your body. If you don't feel tired after your workout, work a little harder. You should not feel like you are punishing yourself when it comes to losing weight.

PROCRASTINATION

I can't tell you how many times I have heard my clients say to me, "I will start my new diet or eating plan tomorrow." The word "procrastination" means "putting off" something we could do right now, today. Our brains are wired to respond to immediate threats and it is more difficult to generate any sense of urgency about something in the future. In other words, it is easier to enjoy that piece of cake right now than think about what you will look in a bathing suit next summer.

We are all guilty of procrastinating at one time or another but there are many of us who procrastinate so much it has a negative effect on our life. You might have a fear of failure or success and perhaps low self-esteem. If you don't overcome procrastinating, it can lead to lost opportunities, no meaning or joy in your life, no satisfaction or achievements. It can cause chronic anxiety and even failure in our relationships.

When it comes to weight loss, procrastination can manifest through our thoughts such as "I don't have time to go to the gym today" or "someone brought dessert into work today so I will start my diet tomorrow." We all know what we should do. Find the time to buy healthy food, prepare it, and exercise. Break down projects into smaller steps and figure out how much time you need to get it done. Taking smaller steps is often a better way to overcome procrastination. Add some dedication and a little self-examination, and successful weight loss is possible.

Do you procrastinate? If you do and are feeling a bit frustrated, it is most likely due to a fear of failure, stress, feeling overwhelmed or not motivated. Increasing your awareness of your feelings is first step in conquering those feelings. If you are procrastinating over your eating plan, it might be that your goals are not appropriate for you. Address your procrastination by giving yourself some structure in your life that is measurable, realistic and attainable. Be patient. Reward yourself for small accomplishments. You can do it.

EVALUATING CHANGES: ANOTHER PHYSICAL ASSESSMENT

Evaluating the changes in your physique and tracking your progress is a critical part of your long-term goals when it comes to losing weight. Evaluating your weight loss along the way can help you stay motivated and encourage you to keep going with your eating plan and exercise program. However, there is more involved in evaluating your weight loss besides simply stepping on the scale. Relying only on what the scale says does not provide the full picture. We can keep track of your progress with the following assessments:

Weigh Yourself – Weighing yourself on a consistent basis, such as the same time one day of each week is a great baseline, especially if you have a lot of weight to lose. However, if you are trying to lose five pounds, you must know that body composition and hydration can affect your weight by as much as two pounds. Don't get discouraged. Weighing yourself is okay as long as we use it conjunction with other methods of measurement.

Use A Tape Measure To Take Circumference Measurements — Measure the circumference of the arm, forearm, waist, hips, and thigh and record the results. The American College Of Sports Medicine recommends repeating each measurement two to three times and recording the average of those measurements. Measurements should be taken once a month and will provide a good look at how your body is changing. Waist measurements provide a good indication of health threats such as diabetes, abnormal body fat levels, metabolic syndrome, and high blood pressure.

Use Fat Calipers To Measure Body Fat Percentage — The most accurate way to measure your body fat is hydrostatic weighing; however, it is quite expensive and not available to everyone. A trained professional can measure your body fat using fat calipers once a month.

Take Progress Photos — Instant photos can be taken with your cell phone or instant camera once a month while wearing clothes that clearly show your shape. Photos will help gauge the changes in your physique, especially when you are focused on gaining muscle and losing body fat. Most likely, you look at yourself in the mirror every day and do not notice subtle changes. Progress photos will reflect those changes when they are taken on a monthly basis.

Pay Attention To How Your Clothes Fit — You may notice your pants are getting a bit baggy, or your wedding ring seems loose on your finger. You might go shopping and notice you can now wear a size smaller — how exciting! It's always fun to acknowledge changes and treat yourself to a new outfit.

Body Mass Index (BMI) — Is a person's weight in kilograms divided by the square of your height in meters. A high BMI can be an indicator of high body fat and a low BMI can be an indicator of having too little body fat. BMI is a screening tool but is not a diagnostic tool for your health. Bone is denser than muscle and twice as dense as fat, so a person with strong bones, good muscle tone, and low fat will have a high BMI. Health-conscious individuals who work out a lot tend to find themselves classified as overweight with a high BMI.

FOOD: THE UPGRADE

There is the old saying that if you give a man a fish, he will eat for a day — but if you teach him how to fish, he will eat forever. This is why a lot of weight loss plans that require you to rely on frozen or prepared "diet" food don't work over the long haul. It's worth the effort to prepare your own food when possible and always plan ahead. It will taste so much better and really won't take much more effort once you get started.

There is truly no one-size-fits-all diet: I want you to learn how to properly nourish your mind, body, and soul according to your needs, with a structure that works. Our weight loss goals are all going to be different, as well as our caloric intake. The nutrients we get in each meal and snack are the common core, and I've provided you an extensive list for you to use to make your meal plan for the week.

For the bigger meals, you want to use the Food Exchange List to balance whole grains, fruit servings, protein servings and fat servings. For snacks, a whole grain and a dairy/fat serving seem to work well for most people in terms of staying energized and full, but you can experiment with what is satisfying to you. The sample guide only mentions vegetable servings at lunch and dinner, but I encourage a handful of non-starchy vegetables with every snack and meal.

It is easy to make a plan using the resources here, but if you want more guidance, FerrignoFIT.com offers the services of professional nutritionists to create personalized meal plans. Whether you create it yourself or have one created for you, you will be following nutritionally sound principles that work for weight loss and maintenance for life.

I have personally been successful on this meal plan, created by the Academy of Nutrition and Dietitians, along with my clients, because it allows you to pick and choose what you want to eat in each category, according to what you're craving. The Food Exchange List educates you about what foods fall into each category and allows you to get creative putting the different categories together.

You won't get bored. You're always in control. There might be food on the exchange list you haven't tried or have ever thought about trying in the past. I encourage you to try at least one new food from each list when you plan your meals on every upgrade/ FITamentalist day. You just might surprise yourself.

As an example, since I follow a version of this plan, here is a breakfast I might have:

2 Whole Grain Servings: 1 slice whole-wheat toast and ½ cup of oatmeal

1 Protein Serving: 2 egg whites

1 Fat Serving: 1 teaspoon of butter

If I'm especially hungry, I might substitute ¼ cup of almonds for the butter. This isn't a trendy diet where all you can eat is watermelon one day and then you eat nothing but almonds and milk the next. It is balanced according to your needs, structured to keep you well-nourished and satisfied. It is also flexible to give you plenty of options to be creative and adjust according to your mood. Once you start following the food exchanges, you'll find that it isn't complicated either.

Now, you might look at this list and think… what is the combo for pizza or chocolate cake? I have never understood the obsession with a "cheat day." Cheating has a negative connotation: it means keeping secrets. Cheating implies you're doing something wrong or "sneaking" to be deceptive, somehow. You know how I feel about that.

Do not hide or avoid feelings and fears by eating. It's okay to reward yourself when you are consistent.Let's flip the dialogue: if you have earned it, consider giving yourself a "treat meal" or "splurge meal" once a week if it helps keep you on track.

FOCUS: Set your goals for your food upgrade based on your journal observations. Where do you need to make changes? What is realistic for you?

INVEST: Choose an appropriate meal plan for the coming week.

TAKE ACTION: Buy the food you will need for your meals. Schedule time to make sure you can stick to your plan. Challenge yourself to try a few new foods. Now get ready to take all the information you have gathered and move forward with your Reset.

CLIENT STORY: RITA

Rita came to me in an electric wheelchair with type 2 diabetes and rheumatoid arthritis. At 59, 5'4", and weighing 339 pounds, she admitted being in constant pain, emotionally and physically. She came to me with the goal of no longer being dependent upon a mobility device or using daily painkillers.

Rita was from the South and struggled with weight her whole life. She grew up eating fried chicken, biscuits, and heaping helpings of pie and cake every night for dessert. At 9, she weighed 184 pounds, and on her wedding day, wore a size 24 wedding dress.

She had gone through eight at-home nurses and fired them all after looking to them for guidance with food education, but instead getting hearty portions of pasta and grilled cheese sandwiches. Her weight kept going up until the day her son, Duke, called in late August of 2009. Her son had decided to get gastric bypass surgery because at 26 he was 364 pounds at 5'11". Rita had a complete breakdown, because she realized she was to blame for his eating habits.

Before that day, Rita was at the point where she was considering moving into an assisted living facility.She was furious with her son at first, that he would take the easy way out and mutilate his body to lose weight. After a few days, her anger turned from her son onto herself and the liters of sodas in the house, the cakes and cookies in cabinets, and the ice cream in the fridge. She threw it all out and called her son back. They made an agreement to partner up and do it the right way.

Simply by limiting their sugar intake, the pounds started dropping off. Duke and Rita joined the local YMCA and swam for 30 minutes, 4 days a week. After a few months, they came to me to consult with them about proper nutrition and to educate them about the cardio/weight room. I had them step up their workout by adding the treadmill starting four days a week for 20-minute sessions that included light weight training and stretching. Rita had not exercised in years and she admitted at first that it was hard to make herself get on that treadmill, but seeing Duke walk next to her and give her a big high five when he saw her struggling was motivation enough for her to keep going.

After two consistent years of weight training, spinning, and Zumba classes, Duke and Rita became closer than ever. Both lost over 130 pounds and have stayed consistent with their weight loss. They kept their faith in the Lord and take each day as a blessing and a gift. Losing the physical and emotional weight they had been carrying around for years opened the door to new opportunities. Rita and Duke said yes to events they were too embarrassed to attend before. Duke got married in 2013 and Rita ditched her house and traveled on a boat to see the world for a year.

THE
RESET PLAN
– WORKBOOK –

LET'S BEGIN

During this program, you will track and record your body measurements every seventh day. For the body measurements, you are going to measure your height to waist ratio as well as waist to hip ratio. You will measure your height and weight with a measuring tape to do this. Your waist size should be less than half of your height. For example if you are 5'2" feet tall (62 inches) the circumference of your waist should be less than 31 inches.

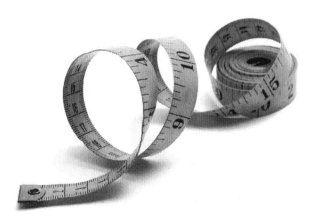

To get your hip to waist measurement, you will measure each and then divide your hip measurement with your waist measurement. Compare your findings with the chart (see next page) and keep track in your journal so you can watch these numbers change. Body measurements are a more accurate gauge of fitness and change than measuring your BMI.

BODY MEASUREMENT

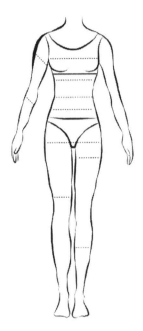

My bust is _____ inches
My upper arm is _____ inches
My chest is _____ inches
My waist is _____ inches
My Forearm is ____ inches
My Midway is _____ inches

My Hips are ____ inches

My Thighs are____ inches

My Knee is ____ inches

My Calves are ____ inches

Week:_____

Total weight:_____ pds

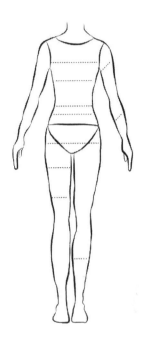

YOU ARE AN ATHLETE AND A *FIT*AMENTALIST

Now that you are an athlete and a FITamentalist, your mindset should be centered on improving your ability to achieve your health and weight loss goals. Expanding on what you have learned expands your understanding of yourself in the process of achieving your desired outcome. Ask yourself:

"Is anything holding me back?"

"What is it about me that I keep on making the same mistake?"

"What am I not aware of that I need to know?"

As you progress in your weight loss journey and learn more, it makes you realize how much you have to learn about yourself and being successful in achieving your weight loss goals. Make a commitment to being open to new information and new ways to lose weight and be healthy.

*FIT*AMENTALIST WEEK 1:

FOCUS: Assess your physical and mental health. Envision your best self.

INVEST: Make a doctor's appointment. Locate or purchase a tape measure and take some key body measurements

SELFIE "BEFORE" SHOTS: Take front, right, and left — and back, if possible.

TAKE ACTION: Put your scale away. Check a nagging project off your to-do list.

YOUR F.I.T. Goals

1. The workouts begin. Beginner? Keep aiming for the 10k step range and be at least in the 8k range at this point. If you reached 10k, begin improving your time and take note. Begin your resistance training workouts.

2. Stay consistent with your journaling/social media.

3. When you wake up it's important to eat within an hour of waking

up. Before you do that you are going to drink an 8oz (Pub Glass) of water with lemon, "breaking the fast"

4. Learning about the origin and effects of HFCS and artificial sweeteners.

5. Remember the importance of sleep.

6. Your water intake should be up from 8-10 Pub Glasses a day. Have a glass of water with every meal or snack.

7. Begin meditation this week. Focus on cutting down stress to reduce its negative effects on the body.

8. When choosing proteins and vegetables make sure you're picking high fiber and colorful foods.

9. Only eat at the dining room or kitchen table. Completely stop eating standing up or while distracted by TV, work, or your phone.

10. Freeze or put away leftovers immediately so you do not overeat.

*FIT*AMENTALIST DAY: Upgrade Week 2

1. Measure and document.

2. Meal preparation.

3. Pick a recipe from Ferrigno FIT you are going to make this week.

4. Pick a FITness sponsor.

5. If it's not on your Food Exchange List, donate, give away, or throw it away.

6. Daily self-talk dialogue and personal mantra.

7. Journal and share your mantra on social media.

The second week of *The Reset Plan* asks you to begin following a flexible, nutritionally-sound eating plan that reduces the amount of sugar you consume and to use the results of last week's journaling to begin to address your relationship with food. Do you always give up your power to things you can't control in the moment? When do you not trust yourself with food? What time of the day and in what scenario are you most vulnerable with food?

Food doesn't have feelings, but you do. Food is not a friend. It's time to learn how to eat according to our goals. Maybe it's not the food you can't trust; instead, is it possible that you don't trust your feelings so you avoid them by eating? Running away from your feelings is a race you will never win. This particular excuse or lie, while very common among my clients, may not speak to every reader. That's okay. It is also a jumping off point for strategies for healthy eating on *The Reset Plan* that will be relevant to everyone.

REVIEW OF PHASE 1: DAY 1-6

This is auditing your food, feelings, and the people around you. I want you to journal and write down your eating and feelings so you become mindful, not ashamed. During this time I don't encourage you to tell people about your new lifestyle. This is *your* time to observe your feelings, the people who support you, the way you speak to yourself, and how you react to anxiety, anger, and identifying what frightens you. I want you to remember to not think of this as a 66-day program, but as a program that has 66 days in it — and that it's one day at a time we need to focus on. You need to concentrate on breaking habits instead of focusing on the number that appears on a scale.

These phases are going to be every 6 days and the upgrade day will always be every 7th day throughout the 66-day program.

Make sure the 7th day is a day where you have at least 3 hours to give to yourself. This day will become your **"FITamentalist" Day**. A day of rest, physically, but also of gains — mentally *and* physically. You are preparing for the next phase ahead. On this 7th day I want you to grocery shop and continue to upgrade your food choices by bringing back the basics. Don't plan this for a day that is hectic for you. If Sunday is the best day to meal prep do it. If it's Wednesday, then great! That's your FITamentalist day.

On the 7th day when you meal prep/grocery shop for the week ahead I want there to be an upgrade. Each week I want you to progress and get cleaner with the ingredients in your food.

Have You Cleaned Out Your Cabinets?

Ditch anything that has more than 5 ingredients on the label and/or anything you can't pronounce. Begin looking for these ingredients:

- Hydrogenated Oils
- High Fructose Corn Syrup

- Monosodium glutamate (MSG)
- All artificial sweeteners (Stevia, Splenda, Aspartame, etc.)
- Anything with food coloring, i.e. Red #40
- Any label that says artificial or food product

Make sure you ditch the following in your cabinet:

- Soda
- Sugar-free anything
- Canned soups
- Plastic-wrapped bread
- Microwave dinners
- Tortillas

Add To Your Kitchen

Focus on more vegetables, including frozen and non-starchy vegetables. Pay attention to your 5 senses. Your tastes are going to change throughout these phases and the 66 days. They are going to be altered by you upgrading them. We are going to simplify them and bring you back to the feeling of tasting these foods for the first time — really smelling them for the first time and enjoying that sensation for the first time. We are not depriving but rather filling the void of deprivation you have had yo-yo dieting all these years. We are going to add back, not take away, and discover your senses again. It's time to upgrade your palate.

Self-Talk Dialogue

Create a self-talk dialogue for yourself, one you will say every morning and one that will be inspiring enough to keep you on track and remind you you're worth it when you don't feel like it. I am *not* a morning person. I was always a grump waking up and used the excuse of "I *need* my coffee before I can function." If I ran out of coffee it could possibly ruin my day.

When I began my morning mantras, my dynamic changed. I wake up thankful and check in with all my friends and loved ones who no longer have a day to spend on this planet. I say my personal mantra to get focused with my day. I notice it helps a lot when I have scheduled a morning workout or had a late night, the night before, to not allow me to make excuses and stay focused on my daily goals.

Have You Bought A Journal?

You can find inexpensive ones at Target, T.J. Maxx, and/or Wal-Mart. Wherever you buy it, find one with a cover that is inspirational to you — mine says "Be Your Own Hero." I want you to write in it:

- Before every meal
- Anytime you feel anxious
- Anytime you're having a craving

Keep these questions in your mind: Am I hungry? Why am I hungry? How much water have I had? Is my environment affecting my hunger? If I eat this, will it send me down an endless, mindless spiral? Regardless, throughout the day, if you write for 20 minutes or 2 minutes, it's important to track the date, time and what you are feeling. I want you to:

FOCUS: On feelings

INVEST: Time, date, and consistency

TAKE ACTION: Write it down

Get Creative

Find ways to get creative with walking up stairs at work for a bathroom break. Begin walking 10-15 minutes a day, hula-hoop, and start finding activities that you like. Get creative with your office: how many steps can you walk a day? Experts will mention that the goal is 10k steps a day. At this point in my life I have surpassed that. I started with 4k steps I now far surpass 10k steps a day. I suggest getting a pedometer and tracking your steps. I found tracking made it a fun game for me. However many steps you take a day, have a goal to begin adding anywhere from 250-400 steps a day to get consistent with the 10k a day mark.

Learning *The Reset Plan's* Food Portion Pyramid

Learn the food pyramid and exchange list. I have listed 4 different caloric and lifestyle suggestions. During these six days, begin implementing them into your meals. Investing in a grill, salad spinner, rice cooker, and Tupperware are all great things to consider. These items are not necessary, but if you have a busy, non-stop lifestyle, it will save you time and anxiety in the long run.

THE RESET PORTION PLAN

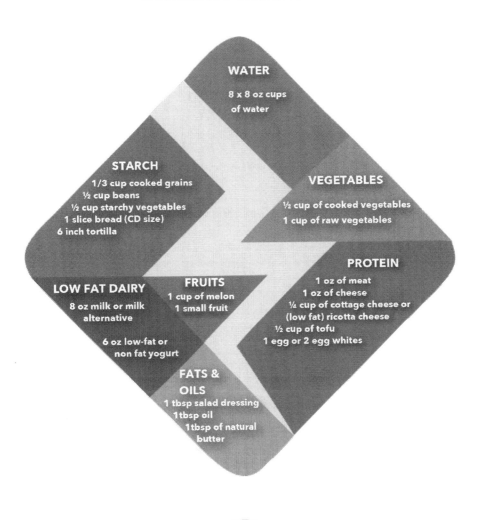

Pick a project in your house/car/office you have been delaying tackling. Mine would be my closet that always gets messy when friends and family come over. Every time people come over I throw all of my extras, to clean up my space, in my hall closet. Days/weeks will pass and I always promise myself will organize, but then make the excuse that I have no time to do it. **Every week during this 66-day period, you are going to work on a project you have been slacking on and finish it.**

Focus On:

- Creating a mantra that works for you
- Notice your feelings and the way you talk to yourself — be present with your 5 senses
- Identifying stress patterns
- Adding steps a day to your routine
- Meal plan and implementing meals
- Wake up and drink water with lemon before breakfast
- Not skipping breakfast

Invest In:

- Learning what products need to be taken out of your meals
- Rice cooker
- Salad spinner
- Tupperware
- Food cooler
- Down sizing your plates and bowls
- Buying a pedometer
- Consulting a doctor

Take Action:

- Getting to know the perimeter at your grocery store
- Answer questions before every meal
- Complete a house project
- Write daily in your food journal
- Prep meals for the week ahead
- Track your daily steps
- Clean out your cabinets

- Add in vegetables
- Eating breakfast every day this week

PHASE 2: DAYS 8-22
UPGRADE DAYS 14 AND 21

- Make dinner the most important meal of the day, both for the emotional factor and for the importance of limiting your carbohydrates at night.
- Use the cooler you hopefully invested in and take refrigerated snacks with you when you go out. You won't feel desperate to eat and you won't be snacking pre-packaged items loaded with sugar or turkey jerky at the nearest 7-11 that's loaded with sodium.
- Cut down on the "white zombies": salt, table sugar, and artificial sweeteners.
- Grab a pair of pants, skirt, and/or shorts that are tight on you and bring them out where you can see them daily.
- Prepare to give up artificial sweeteners and calorie filled drinks by phase 3.
- No eating out these two weeks – but if you must, look over the menu. Know your food chart.
- Review the daily activities that burn calories.
- Next house project you are working on and finishing up. If it's a bigger one, use the two weeks as a goal, a smaller one – one completed each upgrade day.
- Play with your food. Spice it up instead of adding the table salt.
- Fill your freezer, not your cabinets. Grab ziplock bags, buy in bulk, and chop it up. If healthy foods are already prepped, you're more likely to reach for them.

Understanding Yourself

You are going to spend this week auditing your food, your feelings, your exercise, and the people around you. You need a journal to record your observations. If you don't have something around the house you want to use, you can find inexpensive ones at any stationery, office supply, or super-store. Wherever you buy your journal, I want you to find one with a cover that is inspirational to you.

Leave the first five pages of your journal blank for now. You will eventually use these to record the numbers from your blood work and physical, along with any notes or suggestions from your doctor. There is also a place here in the workbook for you to record these results. These are your starting points and your benchmarks. I know it can take time to book an appointment, but ideally you will have some results during the first weeks of this process.

Below are three columns: LUST, LOVE, and INDIFFERENT Write down ten foods under each column that makes you feel the corresponding emotion. As your relationship with food changes in the coming weeks, it's going to be interesting to watch.

LUST	LOVE	INDIFFERENT

Track your biweekly measurements. Take them this week and then again every other week on your upgrade day. Many people find that tracking these measurements is more telling, and more satisfying, than tracking your overall weight on the scale.

Questions To Consider:

- Did you notice patterns in the times of day or night when you made poor food choices?
- Are there any foods or meals that seem hard for you to "control" yourself around?
- How did you feel about the nutritional profile of the foods that are part of your regular grocery list?
- Can you identify factors in your routines that made it easier or harder to fit in some extra movement?
- How do you feel this week after increasing your movement? Were you sore? Tired? Energized? Happier?
- Do the people who you spend your day with follow healthy lifestyle habits like exercising, and watching what they eat?
- Does your partner follow a healthy lifestyle?
- If you go out and eat more than once a, week do the people you eat with order healthfully?
- If you wanted to be active and go for a hike or the gym, how easy is it to find someone to go with you?
- Do the people you live with bring home foods that could contribute to your weight gain?
- When you look in the mirror are you upset, humiliated or frustrated by what you see?
- When you're tired or feeling run down do you blame it on getting older or your stressful environment?

Blood Chemistry:

YOUR TYPICAL DAY OF MEALS

Wake-Up Time: _____
Breakfast: _____
Mid-Morning: _____
Lunch:_____
Mid-Afternoon: _____
Dinner: _____
Beverages: _____
Anything Before Bed?_____

Medications (these can cause weight gain):

Supplements:

When is the best time of day for you to exercise?

When do you remember yourself being at your healthiest?

Questions And Concerns:

TAKE THIS SURVEY:

Why do I want to lose weight?

Are my goals achievable?

What stopped me from my goal before?

What are your self-sabotages? Name them:

What physical activity do you enjoy doing? If it's been a while, think back to when you were a kid.

What would you do and how would you act if you were at your ideal weight right now?

How and where do you usually eat your food? What does the environment feel like? How do you feel in that environment?

Notes:

TRIFECTA
Your Challenge Begins

6-Day FOCUS: Mentality leading up to your Lifestyle Change
30 Days Of Food And Workouts: INVEST
30-Day Workouts: TAKE ACTION

"FOCUS" – TO DOs for the next 6 days:

- Consult a doctor, get bloodwork done, and learn your blood type
- Ditch the scale
- Plant-rich food – cleaning out the liver and intestines (i.e. parsley or chlorophyll)
- Dopamine
- Vitamin D
- Thinking about how you got "here" feeling out of control
- Measure and take pictures of yourself
- Begin to record what you are eating, the feelings you have when you are eating and the environments you eat in.
- Notice how many times you mindlessly eat and/or eat while watching TV or while distracted.
- Take notice about how much sugar you are taking in.
- Think about what activities you enjoy doing. Think back to being a kid.
- Start listening to yourself and track the way you talk about yourself.
- Begin noticing every time you make an excus.
- Begin noticing how many times you say "yes" when you want to say "no."
- Drink a half a gallon of water a day, as well as starting and ending your day by drinking water (hot or cold) with lemon/lemon juice.
- Find one mantra (word) that will inspire you on this journey and begin to visualize what you want to take from the next 60 days.
- Collect motivational memes, quotes, and pictures each of the next 6 days.
- Begin working daily on your posture.

- Begin identifying who in your life fills you and who drains you.
- Begin grocery shopping with cash only.
- Pick the meal plan that best suits your goals ahead.
- Take OUT one food item you know is not good for you from your diet.

"INVEST" – 30 Days

- Take progression pictures and measurements.
- Check in with your doctor.
- Start saying your mantra 6x daily.
- Place your inspirational quotes, pictures and memes in your house, car, and office space.
- Master your food chart. Print it, post it in your kitchen and carry it with you for the next 30 days.
- Limit your alcohol and coffee intake .
- Clean out your cabinets and invest in Tupperware.
- Throw out any processed foods and items that have an ingredient you can't pronounce.
- Always have a list when you grocery shop and stick to the perimeter.
- Pick a meal prep day (*The Reset Plan* day) that works for you.
- Begin taking: multivitamins, probiotics and omegas daily. (For some, anti-inflammatories will be suggested.)
- Find a community/friend that keeps you accountable.
- Relearn the meaning of exercise.
- Start moving for 25-35 minutes daily; include bands and/or light weights during your workouts.
- Internalize the importance of *The Reset Plan.*
- Identify any trauma, especially related to food and eating habits.
- Avoid dehydration.
- Understand how your hormones may affect this process.
- Learn tools to get back your control.
- Learn the correct form for exercising and be conscious of food fads.
- Get to know your heart rate.
- Only eat sitting down.

- Put a dollar in a jar every time you make an excuse.
- No eating out more than once a week.
- Look up the menu before you go to the restaurant.
- Eat before you go out.
- Establishing one cheat meal a week... not a whole day.
- Turn off your cell phone and the TV during dinner.
- Begin getting creative with your leftovers.
- Ditch the salt for other spices, begin shopping with cash.
- Take pictures of your meals and share with your community.
- Be clear what a serving size is.
- Know the manufacturer of everything you eat.
- Buy yourself a nice workout outfit.
- Get to know the Glycemic Index and be able to identify the difference between simple and complex carbs.
- Begin getting your finances in order.

"TAKE ACTION" – Next 30 Days

- Take progression pictures and measurements.
- Check in with your doctor.
- Begin getting detailed with your body parts; names of each.
- Workout 35-55 minutes 5x a week and program with the weights or resistance bands.
- Have a post workout you enjoy? Have you stayed consistent with your stretching and vitamin intake?
- Master your Heart Rate Zone during exercise.
- Have 3 class schedules and options (indoor and outdoor).
- Know the differences between good fats and bad fats.
- Cook at least 1 new recipe a week.
- Know how to take leftovers and make another meal from them.
- Work out with compound movements.
- When you do eat out, set the bar by ordering first.
- Remove one excuse from your life.
- Be conscious of how you feel while you are cooking and eating.

- Pinpoint when you have anxiety and when you second guess yourself.
- Examine what you tolerate.
- Learn facts and details about muscle and why it weighs more than fat.
- Learn what HIIT workouts are and continuing to advance your progression.
- Get rid of any clothes that don't fit.
- Reward yourself with a new outfit, massage, or manicure; not food.
- Have a list of what you will and won't tolerate.
- Pay it forward and bring on someone you are now mentoring.
- Be clear about the healthiest meal options at restaurants.
- No longer eat at fast food chains.
- Maintain your active presence online.
- Educate yourself about plateaus and how to work through them.
- Write a workout and meal plan for yourself if you will be traveling.
- Make peace with the past.
- Be clear about consequences when ditching your goals.
- Recognize and write down any anxiety you have about the program so you can face it and conquer it.
- Begin giving back and sharing what you have learned about yourself on all levels.
- Identify the next habit and excuse to break for the next 66 days.

We are going to implement all of these together, but for the first 6 days of this 66-day F.I.T journey I want to begin with Focus: focus on your mentality towards your thought process and relationship everyone and everything in your life.

66-DAY PROGRAM

FOCUS
First 6 Days:

- Cut out the 3 White Zombies that make you feel lethargic while you're alive and will eventually drag you to your grave: iodized salt, refined sugar, and artificial sweeteners.

- Wake up and drink 8oz of water with lemon.
- 10-20 minutes of walking a day
- Challenge yourself to finding ways to get 10k steps in a day. (Taking the stairs to use the bathroom on another floor at work, parking far away from where you are going, etc.)
- Buy a pedometer or add an app to your phone.
- Buy a journal and begin to write down how you feel throughout the day. Track the day and time when you begin feeling: Anxiety? Cravings? Dehydrated? Stressed?
- Clean out your cabinets. If you can't pronounce the ingredients on the label or can't grow it, then ditch it.
- Counting calories is good to do but you also need a balance of carbohydrates and fats with the *Reset's* Meal Plans.
- Buy spices to replace the salt. Keep the flavor but ditch the sodiumm
- Invest in Tupperware: 8-10 glass pieces.
- Clean your shelves of big bowls and plates; use light colors and child size bowls/plates

7th Day: Meal Prep Day
This will continue to be your prep day every week. Make sure you pick a day that works for you.

- Grocery shopping tips
- Ditching detoxes, preservatives and pre-packaged anything
- I am going to include 6 different recipes that include a lot of the same ingredients for lunches and dinners and also provide 3 for breakfasts. You have a variety of choices with the *Reset's* Meal Plan and Food Exchange list
- Saying goodbye to diets
- Eating 5 times a day – that includes 3 meals and 2 snacks
- Snack ideas of 100 calories or less:
    - Handful of nuts
    - Red pepper slices and hummus

- Greek yogurt and berries
  - Nut butter and apple
  - Cheese and Turkey or other meat slices
  - Hard-boiled eggs
- Continue to journal
- Check in with your posture daily
- Explanation of ingredients; omegas, vitamins, nutrients
- Why dinner is the most important meal of the day

INVEST

Phase 1 (4 weeks) – Adjustment

- Make a playlist/book on tape
- Buy a calendar/whiteboard
- Have a mantra(s)
- No eating out the first two weeks
- Try to avoid salt – but if you're going to have salt, begin to make the adjustments and use Himalayan Pink Salt
- No table sugar
- 64oz of water a day
- Accept that artificial sweeteners are *out*, for good.
- Think in color
- Breaking habits
- Importance of a FIT sponsor
- Work out with bands and cardio Monday-Wednesday-Friday for 40 minutes.

WORKOUT COMBINATIONS:

Level 1 – Arms:
    A. 15 WALL PUSH-UPS
    B. 10 OVER HEAD SHOULDER PRESS
    C. 10 HAMMER CURLS
    D. 15 AIR PUNCHES

Level 1 – Legs/Core
A. 15 SQUATS
B. BRIDGES (30 SECOND HOLD)
C. 10 WALKING LUNGES
D. MOUNTAIN CLIMBERS (30 SECONDS)

Level 1 – All-Over Body Work
A. JUMPING JACKS (30 SECONDS)
B. CRUNCHES (30 SECONDS – 1 MIN)
C. PLANK (30 SECONDS)
D. FLUTTER KICKS (30 SECONDS)

Level 1 – Chest/Shoulders/Back
A. DUMBBELL FLAT BENCH PRESS
B. UPRIGHT DUMBBELL ROWS
C. DUMBBELL SHRUGS
D. DUMBBELL SIDE BEND

LEVEL 1 — 3 SETS OF EACH

***REST IN BETWEEN SETS 2 MIN

LEVEL 1 —3 SETS
LEVEL 2 — 4 SETS
LEVEL 3 – TEST YOUR TIME AND GO UP TO 5 SETS

***REST IN BETWEEN SETS 2 MIN

Level 2 – Arms
A. 15 DUMBBELL SQUAT THRUSTERS/OVERHEAD PRESS
B. 15 BICEP PREACHER CURLS
C. 15 WEIGHTED AIR PUNCHES
D. JUMP ROPE (1 MIN)

Level 2 – Legs/Core
A. 15 JUMP SQUAT
B. 15 BODY WALKING LUNGE
C. ONE LEG BRIDGE HOLDS (1 – 2 MINUTE HOLD)
D. BUTT KICKS (1 MIN)

Level 2 – All-Over Body Work
A. HIGH KNEES

B. FROGGY
C. LEG PULL IN KNEE UP
D. PLANK LEG LIFT

Level 2 – Chest/Shoulders/Back
A. STANDING DUMBBELL LAT RAISES
B. WOOD CHOP
C. SWISS BALL BACK EXT.
D. RENEGADE ROWS

LEVEL 2 — 4 SETS

***REST IN BETWEEN SETS 2 MIN

Level 3 – Mash Up 1
A. 10 LAT RAISES
B. SITTING TWISTS (30 SECONDS)
C. 20 DONKEY KICKS
D. 20 SIDE LEG RAISES

Level 3 – Mash Up 2
A. 10 BENT OVER REVERSE FLYS
B. SUPERMANS
C. SIDE PLANK (30 SECONDS)
D. DUMBBELL DEADLIFT

Level 3 – Mash Up 3
A. 15 UPRIGHT DUMBBELL ROW
B. LUNGE TWIST (1 MIN)
C. JUMP ROPE (1 MIN)
D. SIDE PLANK KNEE KICK

Level 3 – Mash Up 4
A. 15 DUMBBELL WINDMILL
B. 15 INCH WORM /WALK OUT
C. 10 TRICEP DUMBBELL KICK BACKS
D. JACK KNIFE SIT UP (1 MIN)

LEVEL 3 – MIX UP 2 DIFFERENT MASH UPS AND TEST YOUR TIME. THEN GO UP TO 5 SETS.

LEVEL 1 — 3 SETS
LEVEL 2 — 4 SETS
LEVEL 3 — TEST YOUR TIME AND GO UP TO 5 SETS

***REST IN BETWEEN SETS 2 MIN

You can mix and match all of these workouts no matter where you are in your journey. Design your workout based on your day, body part and the time you have. Always test your limits. If you are in pain, they you need to stop. Listen to your body and if it starts to burn early into the sets, you might be on a more advanced level to start.

If you are feeling spontaneous and/or not in the mood to workout use this fun method to get moving! It works for me!

FLIP-A-COIN WORKOUT:

	HEADS	TAILS
1st Flip:	1 min. jog in place	25 jumping jacks
2nd Flip:	20 jump-squats	30 calf raises
3rd Flip:	25 kneeling push-ups	10 push-ups
4th Flip:	45 sec. skipping rope	45 sec. mountain climbers
5th Flip:	40 knee-highs	40 jumping backs
6th Flip:	45 sec. fast squats	45 sec. squat jumps
7th Flip:	50 crunches	20 sit-ups
8th Flip:	25 jumping jacks	1 min. jog in place
9th Flip:	45 sec. burpees	45 sec. butt kicks

REST 15-30 seconds between each exercise, depending on your fitness level.

For example:

- Tuesday-Thursday-Saturday: walk/cardio for 25-30 minutes
- Sunday: Rest day or adjust according to your lifestyle and/or work schedule
- Importance of sleep and rest
- Alcohol is not restricted but not encouraged – alcohol is sugar and stored as body fat. Limit your alcohol intake.

TAKE ACTION:
Phase 2 (4 weeks) Upgrade

- Upgrading your lifestyles and new adjustments
- Make 3 new recipes a week. Upgrade recipes and learn to make leftovers into new meals.
- Make sure you're drinking 64 ounces of water; make "spa water" by filling a pitcher of purified water and adding lemons or limes for flavor and nutrients.
- Upgrade your workouts by adding in weights. 60 min 5x a week – make exercise a part of your daily routine, such as taking the stairs whenever possible.
- Switch to sugar in the raw.
- Make sure you're still avoiding artificial sweeteners.
- Find workouts of your own that you like. Think back to sports you enjoyed playing as a kid and adjust for YOU today.
- Journal your mentality of upgrading all around you
- Start upgrading your wardrobe/overall appearance.
- Think of 5 ways to pay it forward
- Consider becoming a FIT sponsor

Here is the equation that will give you an idea of how to calculate your meal plan:

Your weight in pounds divided by 2.2 = kg

You need 25-30 kcals/kg per body weight (to get kg you divide lbs by 2.2)

For example, if your goal is 120 pounds, you divide 120 by 2.2 (120/2.2) = 54.5kg
54.5 kg x 25 = 1363 kcals
54.5 kg x 30 = 1635 kcals

Therefore, your range should be 1300 - 1600 kcals/day.

1500 Calorie Total Daily Intake
Diabetics & Pre Diabetic

Carbohydrates: 12 servings
Suggested balance: 2 milk servings, 3 fruit servings, 7 whole grain servings

Protein: 6 servings

Fats/Oils: 3 servings

Vegetables: 4 servings minimum

Breakfast

2 Whole Grain servings	
1 Protein serving	
1 Fruit serving	
1 Fat serving	

Lunch

2 Whole Grain servings	
1 Fruit serving	
2 Vegetable servings	
2 Protein servings	
1 Fat serving	
Free Food	

Afternoon Snack

1 Low Fat Dairy serving	
1 Whole Grain serving	

Dinner

2 Whole Grain servings	
1 Fruit serving	
2 Vegetable servings	
3 Protein servings	
1 Fat servings	

1600 Calorie Total Daily Intake

Carbohydrates: 13 servings
Suggested balance: 2 milk servings, 4 fruit servings, 7 whole grain servings

Protein: 6 servings

Fats/Oils: 5 servings

Vegetables: 4 servings minimum

Breakfast

2 Whole Grain serving	1 slice whole wheat toast, 1/2 cup cooked oatmeal
1 Protein serving	2 egg whites scrambled with cooking spray
1 Fat serving	1 Tbsp butter

Morning Snack

1 Fruit serving	1 Apple
1 Low Fat Dairy serving	8oz glass of non fat milk
1 Fat Serving	1/2 Tbsp natural nut butter

Lunch

2 Whole Grain servings	2 slices of whole grain bread
1 Fruit serving	1/2 Banana
2 Vegetable servings	1 cup carrot sticks, 1 cup tomato slices and lettuce
2 Protein servings	2oz of roast turkey
1 Fat serving	2 Tbsp avocado
Free Food	Mustard

Afternoon Snack

1 Low Fat Dairy serving	6oz non fat, plain Greek Yogurt
1 Whole Grain serving	1/4 cup Granola
1 Fruit serving	3/4 cup blueberries

Dinner

2 Whole Grain servings	1/2 large baked potatoes
1 Fruit serving	1/2 cup of Mango
2 Vegetable servings	1 cup cooked green beans, 1 cup mixed greens salad
3 Protein servings	3oz grilled fish
2 Fat servings	1 Tbsp butter, 3 Tbsp Italian Dressing

1700 Calorie Total Daily Intake

Carbohydrates: 14 servings
Suggested balance: 2 milk servings, 4 fruit servings, 8 whole grain servings

Protein: 6 servings

Fats/Oils: 5 servings

Vegetables: 4 servings minimum

Breakfast

2 Whole Grain servings	
1 Protein serving	
1 Fruit serving	
1 Fat serving	

Morning Snack

1 Fruit serving	
1 Low Fat Dairy serving	
1 Fat Serving	

Lunch

2 Whole Grain servings	
1 Fruit serving	
2 Vegetable servings	
2 Protein servings	
1 Fat serving	
Free Food	

Afternoon Snack

1 Low Fat Dairy serving	
1 Whole Grain serving	
1 Fruit serving	

Dinner

2 Whole Grain servings	
1 Fruit serving	
2 Vegetable servings	
3 Protein servings	
2 Fat servings	

1800 Calorie Total Daily Intake

Carbohydrates: 15 servings
Suggested balance: 2 milk servings, 3 fruit servings, 10 whole grain servings

Protein: 6 servings

Fats/Oils: 5 servings

Vegetables: 5 servings minimum

Breakfast

2 Whole Grain servings
1 Protein serving
1 Low Fat Dairy serving
1 Fat serving

Morning Snack

1 Whole Grain servings
1 Fruit serving

Lunch

3 Whole Grain servings
1 Fruit serving
2 Vegetable servings
2 Protein servings
2 Fat serving
Free Food

Afternoon Snack

1 Low Fat Dairy serving
1 Whole Grain serving

Dinner

3 Whole Grain servings
1 Fruit serving
3 Vegetable servings
3 Protein servings
2 Fat servings

THE RESET PLAN

2000 Calorie Total Daily Intake
Gluten Free

Carbohydrates: 16 servings
Suggested balance: 2 milk servings, 4 fruit servings, 10 whole grain servings

Protein: 7 servings

Fats/Oils: 6 servings

Vegetables: 5 servings minimum

Breakfast

2 Whole Grain servings	
1 Fruit serving	
1 Low Fat Dairy serving	
1 Protein serving	
1 Fat serving	

Morning Snack

1 Whole Grain servings	
1 Fruit serving	

Lunch

3 Whole Grain servings	
1 Fruit serving	
2 Vegetable servings	
3 Protein servings	
1 Fat serving	
Free Food	

Afternoon Snack

1 Low Fat Dairy serving	
1 Whole Grain serving	
1 Fat serving	

Dinner

3 Whole Grain servings	
1 Fruit serving	
2 Vegetable servings	
3 Protein servings	
2 Fat servings	

THE RESET PLAN

2000 Calorie Total Daily Intake

Carbohydrates: 16 servings
Suggested balance: 2 milk servings, 4 fruit servings, 10 whole grain servings

Protein: 7 servings

Fats/Oils: 6 servings

Vegetables: 5 servings minimum

Breakfast

2 Whole Grain servings	
1 Fruit serving	
1 Low Fat Dairy serving	
1 Protein serving	
1 Fat serving	

Morning Snack

1 Whole Grain servings	
1 Fruit serving	

Lunch

3 Whole Grain servings	
1 Fruit serving	
2 Vegetable servings	
3 Protein servings	
1 Fat serving	
Free Food	

Afternoon Snack

1 Low Fat Dairy serving	
1 Whole Grain serving	
1 Fat serving	

Dinner

3 Whole Grain servings	
1 Fruit serving	
2 Vegetable servings	
2 Fat servings	

THE RESET PLAN

2200 Calorie Total Daily Intake

Carbohydrates: 19 servings
Suggested balance: 2 milk servings, 5 fruit servings, 12 whole grain servings

Protein: 7 servings

Fats/Oils: 6 servings

Vegetables: 5 servings minimum

Breakfast
2 Whole Grain servings	
1 Fruit serving	
1 Protein serving	
1 Fat serving	

Morning Snack
1 Fruit serving	
1 Low Fat Dairy serving	

Lunch
4 Whole Grain servings	
1 Fruit serving	
2 Vegetable servings	
2 Protein servings	
2 Fat serving	
Free Food	

Afternoon Snack
1 Fruit serving	
1 Protein serving	

Dinner
4 Whole Grain servings	
1 Fruit serving	
3 Vegetable servings	
3 Protein servings	
2 Fat servings	

Bedtime Snack
1 Whole Grain servings	
1 Low Fat Dairy serving	
1 Fat serving	

THE RESET PLAN

2500 Calorie Total Daily Intake

Carbohydrates: 22 servings
Suggested balance: 3 milk servings, 6 fruit servings, 13 whole grain servings

Protein: 7 servings

Fats/Oils: 6 servings

Vegetables: 5 servings minimum

Breakfast

3 Whole Grain servings	
1 Fruit serving	
1 Protein serving	
1 Fat serving	

Morning Snack

1 Fruit serving	1 Whole Grain srvg
1 Low Fat Dairy srvg	1 Fat serving

Lunch

4 Whole Grain servings	
1 Fruit serving	
2 Vegetable servings	
2 Protein servings	
2 Fat serving	
Free Food	

Afternoon Snack

1 Fruit serving	
1 Protein serving	

Dinner

4 Whole Grain servings	
2 Fruit serving	
1 Low Fat Dairy srvg	
3 Vegetable servings	
3 Protein servings	
1 Fat serving	

Bedtime Snack

1 Whole Grain srvg	
1 Low Fat Dairy srvg	1 Fat serving

Disclaimer: *The Reset Plan's Exchange List and Meal Plans are based on material developed by the Academy of Nutrition and Dietetics, American Diabetic Association, and the U.S. Public Health Service. Actual calories consumed may vary depending on food choices, preparation methods, and cooking methods. If you have any questions or concerns regarding proper nutrition, consult a Registered Dietitian at FerrignoFIT.com or TheResetPlanBook.com*

If you want to tweak the meal plan or have a personalized meal plan, which we recommend, you can contact our dietitians at FerrignoFIT.com or TheResetPlanBook.com

Take a look at the following *The Reset Meal Plan and Exchange List* so you will know what you should eat for each meal throughout the day. Each list is divided up by protein, fats, fruits, vegetables, low-fat dairy, starches, and free foods – no doubt, recipe and meal ideas will come to mind.

Get creative with your meal plans and add variety so you and your family can enjoy eating healthy. Make note of the serving sizes or portion sizes for each meal. Utilize measuring spoons and cups, and a scale. However, you can use your thumb to measure one ounce or your palm to measure your protein source.

THE RESET PLAN

PROTEIN

PROTEIN

One portion contains 0 grams of carbohydrate.

Very Lean Meat & Meat Substitutes (about 35 calories per portion)

Cheese (1 gram of fat or less per ounce)	1 ounce
Cottage Cheese (1gram of fat or less per serving)	¼ cup
Egg Substitutes, plain	¼ cup
Egg Whites	2
Fish: cod, flounder, haddock, halibut, trout, lox, tuna (fresh or canned in water)	1 ounce
Game: Duck or pheasant (no skin), venison, buffalo, ostrich	1 ounce
Hot Dog/Sausage (1 gram of fat or less per ounce)	1 ounce
Poultry: Chicken/Turkey (white meat, no skin)	1 ounce
Sandwich Meats (1 gram fat or less per ounce)	1 ounce

Lean Meat and Substitutes (about 55 calories per portion)

Beef: "select" or "choice" cuts of lean beef including round, sirloin, flank steak; tenderloin. Roast (rib, chuck, rump); steak (T-Bone, porterhouse, cubed); ground round	1 ounce
Cheese, grated parmesan	2 Tbsp
Cheese (3 grams of fat or less per ounce)	1 ounce
Cottage Cheese (4.5% fat)	¼ cup
Fish: Catfish, herring, (uncreamed or smoked, salmon (fresh or canned), tuna (canned in oil, drained)	1 ounce
Game: Goose (no skin, rabbit)	1 ounce
Hot Dogs (3 grams of fat or less per ounce	1 ounce
Lamb: roast, chop or leg	1 ounce
Liver, Heart	1 ounce
Oysters	6 medium
Pork: Lean pork including fresh ham, Canadian bacon, tenderloin, centre loin chop	1 Ounce
Poultry: Chicken/Turkey (dark meat, no skin), chicken (white meat with skin), domestic duck or goose (well-drained of fat, no skin)	1 ounce
Sandwich Meats (3 grams fat or less per ounce)	1 ounce
Sardines (canned)	2 medium
Veal: lean chop, roast	1 ounce

243

PROTEIN, MEDIUM & HIGH

MEDIUM-FAT PROTEIN & SUBSTITUTES (75 calories per portion)

Beef: ground beef, meatloaf, corned beef, short ribs, prime rib	1 ounce
Cheese (5 grams of fat or less per ounce) including feta and Mozzarella	1 ounce
Cheese, Ricotta	¼ cup
Egg	1
Fish: Any fried fish product	1 ounce
Lamb: Rib roast, ground lam	1 ounce
Pork: Top loin, chop, boston butt, cutlet	1 ounce
Poultry: Chicken (dark meat with skin), ground turkey or Chicken, fried chicken (with skin)	1 ounce
Sausage (5 grams of fat or less per ounce)	1 ounce
Tempeh	¼ cup
Tofu	4 oz. or ½ cup
Veal: Cutlet (ground or cubed, unbreaded)	1 ounce

High-Fat Meat & Meat Substitutes (about 100 calories per portion)	
Cheese: American, cheddar, Monterey jack, swiss	1 ounce
Hot Dog (beef, pork, or combination) Count as 1 high fat meat plus 1 fat exchange	1 (10/lb)
Hot Dog (chicken or turkey)	1 (10/lb)
Pork: spareribs, ground pork, pork sausage	1 ounce
Sandwich Meats: (8 grams of fat or less per ounce) Including Bologna, pimento loaf, salami	1 ounce
Sausage including bratwurst, Italian, knockwurst, polish, smoked	1 ounce

THE RESET PLAN

VEGETABLES

VEGETABLES

One portion (½ cup cooked or 1 cup raw) contains about 25 Calories and about 5 grams of carbohydrates.

Artichoke
Asparagus
Bean Sprouts
Beets
Broccoli
Brussels sprouts
Cabbage
Cauliflower
Celery
Cucumber
Eggplant
Green Beans
Green Onions
Greens (collard, kale, mustard, turnip)
Leeks

Lettuce
Mushrooms
Okra
Onions
Parsley
Pea Pods
Peppers (all varieties)
Radishes
Spinach
Tomato
Turnips
Water Chestnuts
Watercress
Zucchini

FRUIT

FRUIT

One portion contains about 60 calories and about 15 grams of carbohydrates (the fruit weight includes skin, core, seeds and rind)

Apple	1 small (4oz.)
Apple sauce	½ cup
Apricots (canned)	½ cup
Apricots (fresh)	4 whole (5 ½ oz.)
Banana	1 smalll (4 oz.)
Blackberries	¾ cup
Cantaloupe	1/3 small (11 oz.) or 1 cup cubes
Cherries (canned)	½ cup
Cherries (fresh)	12 cherries (3 oz.)
Figs	2 medium (3 ½ oz.)
Grapefruit	½ grapefruit (11 oz.)
Grapes (small)	17 grapes (3 oz.)
Honeydew	1 slice (10 oz.) or 1 cup cubes
Kiwi	1 fruit (3 ½ oz.)
Mango	½ small (5 ½ oz.)
Nectarine	1 (5 oz.)
Orange	1 small
Papaya (fresh)	½ fruit (8 0z.) or 1 cup cubes
Peach (fresh)	1 medium (4 oz.)
Peaches (canned)	½ cup
Pear	½ large (4 oz.)
Pears (canned)	½ cup
Pineapple (canned)	½ cup
Pineapple (fresh)	¾ cup
Plums	2 small (5 oz.)
Raspberries	1 cup
Strawberries	1 ¼ cup whole berries
Tangerines	2 small (8 oz.)
Watermelon (cubes)	1 slice (13 ½ oz.) or 1 ¼ cup cubes

DRIED FRUIT

Apricots	8 halves
Dates	3
Figs	1 ½
Prunes	3
Raisins	2 tabelspoons

JUICE

Apple Juice	½ cup (4 oz.)
Cranberry Juice	1/3 cup
Grape Juice	1/3 cup
Grapefruit Juice	½ cup
Orange Juice	½ cup
Pineapple Juice	½ cup
Prune Juice	1/3 cup

FAT

FAT

One portion contains about 45 calories and 0 grams of carbohydrates

Monounsaturated Fats

Almonds	6 nuts
Avocado	2 Tbsp
Olives, black	8 large
Olive Oil	1 tsp
Cashews	6 nuts
Mixed nuts (50 % peanuts)	6 nuts
Peanuts	10 nuts
Pecans	4 halves
Peanut butter, natural	½ Tbsp
Sesame Seeds	1 Tbsp
Tahini or sesame paste	2 Tbsp

Polyunsaturated Fats

Margarine	1 Tbsp
Margarine, diet	1 Tbsp
Mayonnaise	1 Tbsp
Mayonnaise, diet	1 Tbsp
Oil (corn, safflower, soybean)	1 Tbsp
Salad Dressing	1 Tbsp
Salad Dressing, reduced fat	2 Tbsp
Seeds: pumpkin, sunflower	1 Tbsp
Walnuts	4 halves

Saturated Fats

Bacon	1 slice
Butter	1 Tbsp
Chitterlings, boiled	2 Tbsp
Coconut, shredded	2 Tbsp
Cream Cheese	1 Tbsp (½ oz.)
Cream Cheese, reduced fat	1 ½ Tbsp (¾ oz.)
Cream, Half & Half	2 Tbsp
Lard	1 Tbsp
Shortening	1 Tbsp
Sour Cream	2 Tbsp
Sour Cream, reduced fat	3 Tbsp

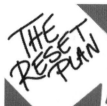

LOW FAT DAIRY

LOW FAT DAIRY

One portion contains about 90-120 calories and about 12 grams of carbohydrates.

Milk, Low Fat (1%)	1 cup (8 oz.)
Milk, Reduced Fat (2%)	1 cup (8 oz.)
Milk, Fat-Free	1 cup (8 oz.)
Milk, Soy (low-fat)	1 cup (8 oz.)
Yogurt*	¾ cup (6 oz.)

(*Plain or sweetened with non nutritive sweetener)

THE RESET PLAN

STARCH

STARCH

One portion contains about 80 calories and about 15 grams of carbohydrate.

Bagel, 4oz.	¼ (1oz.)
Beans & Lentils (cooked)	½ cup (count as 1 starch & 1 very lean meat)
Biscuit, 2 ½" across	½ 6"pita
Bread, Raisin	1 slice
Bun, Hamburger or Hotdog	½ bun
Cereal, cooked	½ cup
Cereal, dry, unsweetened	¾ cup
Chips, baked (tortilla/potato)	5-20 (3/4 oz)
Corn	½ cup
Corn bread, 2" cube	1 (count as 1 starch and 1 fat)
Couscous	1/3 cup
Crackers, animal	8
Cracker, saltine-type	6
English Muffin	½ muffin
Graham Crackers	3 squares
Pancake, 4"across	1 pancake
Pasta, cooked	1/3 cup
Peas, green	½ cup
Plantain	3 cups
Potato, baked with skin	¼ large (3 oz.)
Potato, mashed	½ cup
Pretzels	¾ oz.
Rice (cooked)	1/3 cup
Tortilla (corn)	1 (6" across)
Sweet Potato	½ cup
Squash, winter*	1 cup
(*acorn, butternut, pumpkin)	

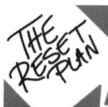

FREE FOODS

FREE FOODS

The following foods are considered "free" foods

Bouillon or broth, low-sodium
Club Soda
Coffee, black
Diet Soda
Drink mixes, sugar free
Garlic
Gelatin Dessert, sugar free
Gelatin, unflavored
Herbs, fresh or dried
Horseradish
Lemon Juice
Lime Juice
Mineral Water
Mustard
Nonstick cooking spray
Spices
Sugar substitutes
Tea
Vinegar
Wine, used in cooking

CROCKPOT COOKING

Cooking food in a crockpot is one of the most efficient and healthy ways to have a great meal waiting for you when you arrive home. Utilizing a wide variety of liquids such as water, vegetable or beef or chicken broth, low-fat gravies, and healthy unsweetened almond milk can ensure a healthy meal in a short amount of time. If you have a pressure cooker, the cooking times are much less than ordinary cooking and as the evaporation created is eliminated, only a small amount of liquid is required.

No matter what you are cooking, the liquids used must completely cover the bottom of the cooker so it will last during the entire cooking time. However, when it comes to cooking stews, soups and puddings, the amount of liquid needed is increased, regardless of the cooking time.

When it comes to cooking solid foods, you should never have the crockpot more than two-thirds full. There must be enough room for the steam or heat to circulate and do its job. Make sure there is enough space between the food and the lid to prevent the steam vent from getting blocked in any way. For liquids, the maximum amount should only be halfway from the base to allow for the liquids to boil.

You might have a favorite recipe you would like to cook in your pressure cooker or crockpot. There might be a basic recipe or something similar with comparable ingredients allowing you to work with the instructions, using your ingredients. If you have a recipe that is cooked traditionally in the oven, take one-third of the normal cooking time for cooking in your pressure cooker or crockpot.

Invest in an immersion blender, as it makes it so much easier to blend the soup recipes into a creamy, smooth texture. It will save you time and energy. If you don't have one, then ladle the soup into a regular blender or food processor and blend slowly. Smaller batches can be done to minimize the risk of splashing.

You will notice that Himalayan Pink Salt is used in the recipes for seasoning. Himalayan Pink Salt is a healthier than regular sea salt and will not elevate blood pressure. It is available at most health food markets and grocery stores in bulk for grinding it fresh with each use.

CROCKPOT RECIPES

SQUASH SOUP WITH CHICKEN AND APPLES
Serves 4
Calories per serving: 228

Making soup in your crockpot is one of the most efficient ways to create a healthy and delicious meal. You can throw all the ingredients in the crockpot in the morning and dinner is ready when you get home. This recipe uses both the green and white parts of leeks. You can always substitute green onions, if needed. The flavor is amazing.

Ingredients:
1 tablespoon of extra-virgin olive oil
1½ cup of chopped leaks or 8 green onions
2 cups of cooked chicken
4 cups of filtered water
4 Honey Crisp or Pink Lady apples – peeled and quartered
3 pounds of butternut squash – peeled, seeded and chopped
1/3 cup of steel-cut oats
2 tablespoons of fresh ginger – minced or 1 teaspoon of ground ginger
1 tablespoon of curry powder
1 teaspoon Himalayan Pink Salt
Fresh Ground Pepper to taste

Directions:
Heat the olive oil in the slow cooker and add the leeks or green onions — sauté for at least one minute before adding the rest of the ingredients. Close the lid and cook for at least 6-7 hours.

Turn OFF the heat. Remove the lid and preferably use an immersion blender to puree the soup to a creamy, smooth texture or until any lumps are gone.
Make sure it is hot before serving and garnish with a dollop of plain Greek yogurt

and chopped walnuts.

Cook's Tip: Roast a bag of chopped walnuts in the oven at 375 degrees for about 10 minutes. Simply spread them out evenly on a cookie sheet. It really does bring out their flavor and adds extra crunch to the soup.

Calories per 1½ cup serving with salad: 228
Calories for soup only: 190

Protein: 4 grams
Fat: 3 grams
Carbohydrates: 42 grams

ITALIAN WEDDING SOUP WITH SIDE SALAD
Serves: 4
Calories per serving: 325

Italian Wedding soup is such a treat and this recipe makes it easy to prepare for you and your family in a crockpot.

Ingredients:
2 tablespoons of extra-virgin olive oil
½ pound of Italian turkey Sausage – removed from the casing
½ pound of ground turkey breast
1 small red onion – diced
½ cup pearl barley
3 garlic cloves or 3 teaspoons of minced garlic packed in olive oil
1 cup of lentils
1 bag of fresh spinach
4 cups of chicken or vegetable broth
½ cup of mild salsa

Directions:
Pour 1 tablespoon of olive oil in the bottom of a large skillet cooker. Mix the turkey meat with the turkey sausage and form turkey balls. Add the turkey meatballs to the skillet and cook. Spoon them into the slow cooker. Add the remaining ingredients and enough chicken broth to cover everything in the slow cooker.

Place the lid on top and slow cook for 6-7 hours.

Cook's Tip: You can substitute chickpeas for the lentils or leave them out altogether. Look for Ranch dressing in the produce section that is made with Greek yogurt; it is less fattening with fewer calories and more protein.

SIDE SALAD

Ingredients:
1 head of Romaine lettuce – chopped
1 Roma tomato – chopped
1 green onion – diced
¼ cup of ranch dressing – preferably Bolthouse brand made from Greek yogurt

Directions:
In a bowl, toss together lettuce, tomato, green onion and dressing – serve immediately.

Calories per 1 cup serving with a side salad: 325
Calories for soup only: 150

Protein: 23 grams
Fat: 12 grams
Carbohydrates: 26 grams

STEAMED LOBSTERS SERVED WITH FRESH ASPARAGUS AND PORCINI MUSHROOM RISOTTO
Serves: 4
Calories per serving: 465

One of the most powerful antioxidants on the planet is found in the shell of lobsters known as Astaxanthin. When a lobster is cooked, the other pigments found in their shell break down, leaving the bright red color that appears on your plate. Cooking lobsters in a slow cooker or crockpot is an excellent and easy way to enjoy them.

Ingredients:

1 bunch of fresh Asparagus – ends broken off

1 tablespoon of extra-virgin olive oil

1 teaspoon of garlic powder

1 cup of white wine or water

4 8-ounce lobster tails

Himalayan Pink Salt and pepper

Directions:

Preheat oven to 375 degrees. Before you are ready to serve dinner, spread asparagus out on a cookie sheet with a lip around the edges. Drizzle olive oil over the top and sprinkle with garlic powder. Season with Himalayan Pink Sea salt and pepper to taste. Bake in the oven for 15 minutes.

Place the lobster tails inside the slow cooker, shell side down. Pour wine or water over all. Secure the lid in place and slow cook for 6-7 hours on low. Remove the lid and season with sea salt.

Cook's Tip: The lobsters will taste delicious whether they are cooked in wine or water. Mushroom risotto can be made ahead of time before the lobsters are cooked.

BROWN RICE MUSHROOM RISOTTO WITH PORCINI MUSHROOMS

Ingredients:

8 cups of low-sodium chicken broth

1 ounce of dried porcini mushrooms

2 tablespoons olive oil

1 red onion – chopped

10 ounces of Portabella mushrooms – chopped

2 cloves of garlic – minced

1½ cups of brown rice

2/3 cup of dry white wine

1/3 cup of Parmesan cheese – grated

Himalayan Pink Salt and pepper to taste

Directions:

In a medium saucepan, bring the broth to a boil. Add the porcini mushrooms and set aside until the mushrooms are tender, about 5 minutes. Keep the broth warm over a very low heat.

In a large saucepan on medium heat, add the olive oil and onions and sauté until tender, about 8 minutes. Add the Portabella mushrooms and garlic. Using a slotted spoon, transfer the porcini mushrooms to a cutting and chop the mushrooms before adding to the saucepan.

Sauté until all the mushrooms are tender and the juices evaporate, about 5 minutes. Stir in the rice and let it brown for a few minutes. Add the wine and cook until the liquid is absorbed, stirring often, about 2 minutes.

Add 1 cup of hot broth; simmer over medium-low heat until the liquid is absorbed, stirring often, about 3 minutes. Continue to cook until the rice is just tender and the mixture is creamy, adding more broth by the ladleful. Stir often, about 30 minutes. The rice will absorb about 6 to 8 cups of broth. Add the Parmesan and season with salt and pepper to taste.

Calories per lobster with risotto: 465

Protein: 31 grams
Fat: 12 grams
Carbohydrates: 48 grams

BAKED TILAPIA WITH SHRIMP SAUCE
SERVED WITH BROWN RICE AND STEAMED BROCCOLI
Serves: 4
Calories per serving: 355

It is possible to cook the tilapia, brown rice and broccoli in a slow cooker all at once for a complete meal that is healthy and delicious. All the flavors blend well together making a delicious, flavored brown rice and broccoli.

Ingredients:
¼ cup of extra-virgin olive oil
¼ cup of whole-grain flour
1 cup of plain almond milk
Himalayan Pink Salt and pepper
Juice of one lemon
1 egg yolk
11/2 cups of cooked shrimp – chopped

1 cup of brown rice
1 head of broccoli – cut into pieces
4 6-ounce Tilapia filets
Parmesan cheese for garnish

Directions:

Heat the olive oil in the bottom of the pressure cooker. Add the flour and milk and mix well. Cook until thickened. Add the sea salt, pepper, egg yolk and cooked shrimp. Stir well. Add the rice and broccoli and place tilapia filets on top of all. Season the filets with fresh ground pepper.

Place the lid on top and cook for 5-6 hours. Sprinkle a tablespoon of grated Parmesan cheese on top of each serving.

Cook's Tip: Any fish will work for you if Tilapia filets are not available.
Calories per serving with fresh broccoli and brown rice: 355

Protein: 26 grams
Fat: 9 grams
Carbohydrates: 23 grams

BAKED SALMON WITH CITRUS TOPPING, NEW RED POTATOES AND SPINACH
Serves: 4
Calories per serving: 375

This classy recipe will impress your guests at your next dinner party. The lemon, lime and orange slices add incredible flavor to the salmon.

Ingredients:
4 6-ounce salmon filets
1 teaspoon of onion powder
Himalayan Pink Salt and pepper to taste
1 lemon – sliced
1 lime - sliced
1 orange – sliced

1 red onion – sliced
4 medium-size new red potatoes
1 16-ounce bag of fresh spinach
2 tablespoons of extra-virgin olive oil
2 tablespoons of sugar-in-the-raw
2 cups of fresh squeezed orange juice
2 tablespoons of cornstarch
¼ cup of soy sauce
¼ cup of apple cider vinegar

Directions:

Season the salmon filets with the onion powder, sea salt and pepper. Arrange the filets in the bottom of the slow cooker. Top with fruit, onion slices, red potatoes and spinach. Mix the olive oil, sugar, orange juice, cornstarch, soy sauce and vinegar in a bowl. Pour over all. Secure the lid and cook for 5-6 hours. Serve immediately.

Cook's Tip: This recipe also work well with other fish filets, however if they are thin, reduce the cooking time by 1-2 minutes, depending on their thickness.

Calories per serving of salmon, 1 potato and ½ cup of spinach: 375

Protein: 18 grams
Fat: 9 grams
Carbohydrates: 15 grams

COD WITH FRESH ASPARAGUS AND SWEET POTATOES
Serves: 4
Calories per serving: 397

Cod is an excellent fish to prepare in a slow cooker. It will absorb any herbs you might use and cooks easily with the asparagus and sweet potatoes.

Ingredients:
4 6-ounce cod filets
1 bunch of fresh asparagus
2 large sweet potatoes – peeled and cut into small squares
2 tablespoons of fresh parsley – chopped
1 cup of white wine

Juice of one lemon
2 garlic cloves – chopped
1 teaspoon of dried oregano
1 teaspoon of paprika

Directions:
Place the cod filets in the bottom of the slow cooker and top with the fresh asparagus and sweet potatoes. Pour the wine and lemon juice over all. Season with Himalayan Pink Salt and pepper – then sprinkle the garlic, oregano and paprika over all. Secure the lid and cook for 5-6 hours.

Serve the cod immediately with asparagus. Pour the wine and lemon juice liquid over all when serving.

Cook's Tip: One tablespoon of fresh oregano works well. For added flavor and crunch, sprinkled toasted almond slivers on top. Vegetable or chicken broth can be substituted for the wine.

Calories per serving: 397

Protein: 16 grams
Fat: 5 grams
Carbohydrates: 27 grams

SIMPLE CHILI SHRIMP WITH BROWN RICE AND MIXED VEGETABLES
Serves: 4
Calories per serving: 347

Cooking shrimp in your slow cooker could not be easier, especially with this simple recipe. Look for chili sauce in the condiment aisle in your local grocery store.

Ingredients:
1 pound of peeled shrimp
1½ cups of brown rice
2 cups of frozen mixed vegetables
1 tablespoon of garlic powder

1 jar of chili sauce

Directions:

Place the shrimp, brown rice and mixed vegetables in your slow cooker. Season with the garlic powder and pour the chili sauce over all. Secure the lid and cook for 5 -6 hours. Serve immediately.

Cook's Tip: These shrimp stand up by themselves as an appetizer or can be served with a side of brown rice and vegetables.

Calories per 4 shrimp, ½ cup of brown rice and ½ cup of vegetables: 347

Protein: 12 grams
Fat: 11 grams
Carbohydrates: 48 grams

COCONUT-CURRY FILETS SERVED WITH WHITE RICE AND PEAS
Serves: 4
Calories per serving: 487

Coconut and curry taste delicious with any kind of fish or shrimp. This recipe is quick and easy and works well for lunch or dinner.

Ingredients:
4 6-ounce white fish filets
½ cup of coconut milk
1½ cups of white rice
2 cups of fresh or frozen peas
2 tablespoons of extra-virgin olive oil
2 Roma tomatoes – diced
1 red pepper – cut into strips
1 red onion – chopped
2 garlic cloves – minced
1 tablespoon of ground ginger
1 teaspoon of ground turmeric
2 tablespoons of ground cumin
1 teaspoon of hot red pepper flakes

½ teaspoon of fenugreek
Himalayan Pink Salt to taste
Juice of one lemon

Directions:
Place the fish, olive oil, red peppers and the remaining ingredients in the slow cooker. Add the spices, rice and peas. Pour the coconut milk over all. Add the tomatoes on top.

Secure the lid and cook for 5-6 hours. Serve immediately with the tomatoes, red peppers and onions on top. Season with salt and sprinkle lemon juice on top of each filet.

Cook's Tip: Frozen fish works well in this recipe. You can also use 2 tablespoons of chopped fresh ginger instead of dried ginger in this recipe.

Calories per serving of shrimp, rice and peas: 487

Protein: 22 grams
Fat: 18 grams
Carbohydrates: 42 grams

MEDITERRANEAN FILETS WITH FINGERLING POTATOES AND CAULIFLOWER
Serves: 4
Calories per serving: 495

You don't need to leave the country to enjoy the Mediterranean flavor in this fish recipe. The tomatoes and capers give this dish a sweet and tart flavor that is quick and easy to prepare.

Ingredients:
4 6-ounce whitefish filets
1 small container of cherry tomatoes
8 fingerling potatoes – washed and dried
1 head of cauliflower – cut into pieces
2 sprigs of fresh thyme leaves or 1 teaspoon of ground thyme

1 cup of vegetable broth
2 tablespoons of pickled capers
1 cup of green olives
1 garlic clove – minced
2 tablespoons of extra-virgin olive oil
Himalayan Pink Salt and pepper to taste
More sprigs of thyme for garnish

Directions:

Place half of the cherry tomatoes, potatoes and cauliflower in the bottom of the slow cooker. Add the fresh thyme and broth. Place the filets on top. Sprinkle the capers, olives and garlic over the fish. Drizzle with olive oil and season with sea salt and pepper to taste.

Secure the lid and cook for 5 – 6 hours. Serve on individual plates and garnish with more cherry tomatoes and fresh thyme sprigs.

Cook's Tip: This recipe works well with salmon too.

Calories per serving of filet, 2 potatoes and ½ cup of cauliflower: 495

Protein: 33 grams
Fat: 12 grams
Carbohydrates: 42 grams

SEAFOOD CHOWDER WITH ROMAINE SALAD TOSSED IN PEANUT BUTTER VINAIGRETTE
Serves: 4
Calories per serving: 395

This recipe is so delicious and easy to make in a slow cooker. It makes a hearty seafood meal all by itself.

Ingredients:
4 6-ounce haddock filets – cut into chunks
6 fingerling potatoes – cut into chunks
1 yellow onion – chopped

1 cup of plain almond milk
½ cup of chicken or vegetable broth
½ cup of plain Greek yogurt
Himalayan Pink Salt and pepper to taste

Directions:
Place the fish chunks, potatoes, onion, almond milk, broth and water in the slow cooker. Secure the lid and cook for 6-7 hours. Open the lid and set the heat to low. Stir in the yogurt and season with sea salt and pepper to taste. Continue to stir until the chowder is thickened. Serve immediately.

Cook's Tip: Haddock is used in this recipe, however any white fish will work. For a healthier recipe, cream is replaced with plain Greek yogurt. It adds protein with less fat for healthier chowder.

PEANUT BUTTER VINAIGRETTE

Ingredients:
In a bowl, whisk together the following ingredients:
¼ cup of apple cider vinegar
1 tablespoon of fresh ground peanut butter
½ teaspoon of ground red pepper
1 teaspoon of Italian herbs
1 teaspoon of garlic powder
½ cup of extra virgin olive oil

Directions:
Place vinegar, peanut butter and spices in a bowl. Whisk in the olive oil until a smooth consistency forms. Toss with Romaine lettuce, chopped tomato and sprinkle salad with 1 tablespoon of grated Parmesan. Enjoy!

Calories per 1½ cup of chowder with Side Salad in Peanut Butter Vinaigrette: 395

Protein: 32 grams
Fat: 7 grams
Carbohydrates: 22 grams

Remember the three columns: LUST, LOVE, and INDIFFERENCE, where you wrote down ten foods under each column that made you feel the corresponding emotion? Your relationship with food has most likely changed over the past few weeks — it will be interesting to see and discuss the changes you have experienced. Are you still lusting, loving or feeling indifferent to those foods?

LUST	LOVE	INDIFFERENT

NAME:

Measurement Weight Loss Chart

Starting Weight: Starting Date:

	Week 1	Week 2	Week 3	Week 4	Week 5	Week 6	Week 7	Week 8	Week 9	Week 10	Week 11	Week 12
Weight												
Weekly Wt. Loss												
Cumulative Wt.												
% of Wt Lost												
Upper Chest												
Bust												
Right Arm												
Left Arm												
Waist												
Hips												
Right Thigh												
Left Thigh												
Weekly Inch Los												
Cumulative In.												

ACKNOWLEDGMENTS

My Family

Thank you first and foremost to my mother **Carla**, who has always believed in me and since day one has given me the strength and support to always be my most authentic self. My father, **Lou**, thank you for giving me the chance to grow up with a man who is loyal, consistent, and showing me the meaning of mental, physical, and spiritual strength. To **my brothers**, I love you and I am proud to be your sister.

The Trifecta

Brie, Corey, and Michelle: Thank you for the endless hours of conversations and realizations, and for helping me with this journey and many others over the years. I truly have learned so much from you three and grown having you kick-ass women in my life.

Topher

Thank you for your endless support emotionally and creatively. You're my rock, Viking, and best friend. I love you.

Tyson

Thank you for your loyalty and for being by my side for the last 11 years. I would have had a lonely decade (plus) without you. Here's to many more.

The Reset Plan Team

I want to give special thanks to my editor and friend **Sherry Granader (sgtotalhealth. com)** for mentoring me through my first book and for her unwavering support. Thank you for helping me put my story and many others' into words.

Julia Todd (@JuliaToddWrites): Thank you for your knowledge and expertise as my go-to editor on the last leg of the book. Thank you for helping me get all my commas in line, input, and vowels in check!

Kim Braniff (@InsideOutNutrition): Thank you for all your support and help with Ferrigno FIT over the years. You are not only a friend and but an amazing dietitian. Thank you for all your input with the nutritional side of the book.

Charlotte Shih (charlotteshih.net): You are a creative rockstar. Thank you for all your hard work designing this book and making it beautiful inside and out.

My Clients

Thank you for helping to inspire this book. Thank you for teaching me every session and being so honest with your truth.

ABOUT THE AUTHOR

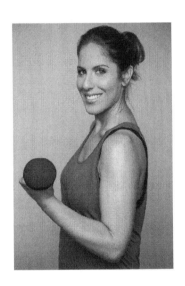

Shanna is a native Angelino. Born and raised in Los Angeles, she essentially grew up living and breathing fitness. Despite being raised in a fitness family (her dad is famed body builder and actor Lou Ferrigno), she had her own weight struggles which inspired her to start Ferrigno FIT, a lifestyle fitness company and to write her first book, *The Reset Plan: Lose the Secrets, Lose the Excuses, Lose the Weight*. Upbeat, fun and accessible, sharing her own personal struggles with weight loss, Shanna will delve into the psychology of shame and food addiction to help you succeed in true health and fitness. Shanna currently lives in Playa Del Rey.

Made in the USA
Columbia, SC
27 July 2021

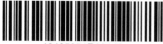
42495851R00148